Nutritional Modulation of Dietary Sugars as a Strategy to Improve Insulin Resistance and Energy Balance in Diabetes

Editor

Paulo Matafome

MDPI • Basel • Beijing • Wuhan • Barcelona • Belgrade • Manchester • Tokyo • Cluj • Tianjin

MDPI

Editor
Paulo Matafome
University of Coimbra
Coimbra, Portugal

Editorial Office
MDPI
St. Alban-Anlage 66
4052 Basel, Switzerland

This is a reprint of articles from the Special Issue published online in the open access journal *Diabetology* (ISSN 2673-4540) (available at: https://www.mdpi.com/journal/diabetology/special_issues/sugar_obesity_diabetes).

For citation purposes, cite each article independently as indicated on the article page online and as indicated below:

LastName, A.A.; LastName, B.B.; LastName, C.C. Article Title. *Journal Name* **Year**, *Volume Number*, Page Range.

ISBN 978-3-0365-8142-2 (Hbk)
ISBN 978-3-0365-8143-9 (PDF)

Contents

About the Editor

Paulo Matafome

Paulo Matafome holds a PhD in Biomedical Sciences (Faculty of Medicine, University of Coimbra, 2012). He is a Physiology Professor at the Coimbra Health School, Polytechnic University of Coimbra. He is also a Researcher at the Coimbra Institute of Clinical and Biomedical Research (iCBR), Faculty of Medicine of the University of Coimbra, and an integrated member of CIBB (research center of the University of Coimbra). He has published 88 research articles (12 as the first author and 22 as the main author) and 4 book chapters, having ∼1950 citations (h factor = 25, Scopus.com). He currently is Associate Editor of several journals and Deputy Editor-in-Chief of *Diabetology*. He has supervised or co-supervised 10 PhD students (4 concluded), 18 MSc students, and 21 BSc Students, coordinating and participating in several national and international research projects. He currently is one of the co-coordinators of the Project PAS GRAS funded by the Horizon program—Cluster Health.

Preface to "Nutritional Modulation of Dietary Sugars as a Strategy to Improve Insulin Resistance and Energy Balance in Diabetes"

Dietary changes toward the increased consumption of Westernised diets and processed food is associated with the increasing prevalence of overweight in young adults and risk of obesity and associated pathologies later in life. The consumption of added sugars contributes to an increased energy density in diet, leading to a positive energy balance, larger waist circumference, and weight gain, increasing the risk of obesity and type 2 diabetes. Moreover, there is a strong association of whole-body and abdominal fat mass with type 2 diabetes, cardiovascular diseases, and cancers. Fat accumulation and body mass index (BMI) are directly proportional to the excessive intake of energy in relation to expenditure, especially from foods rich in fats. Sugars may be divided into two distinct groups: those naturally present and those added to foods. Natural or intrinsic sugars are naturally present in foods, such as fruit sugar (fructose), vegetables, honey, and sugars from dairy products (galactose and lactose). Added sugars are a large group of mono- and di-saccharides that go into foods during processing, preparation, or at the table, with the objective of sweetening, increasing food palatability and shelf life, improving texture, inhibiting the growth of microorganisms in high concentrations, providing functional structures, or increasing accessibility. They are mostly found in sugary drinks, pastry products, cookies, fruit juices, energy drinks, nectars, fruit juices from concentrate, white bread, and breakfast cereals. The impact of dietary sugars on the pathophysiological mechanisms of type 2 diabetes and its complications is not entirely understood.

Paulo Matafome
Editor

diabetology

MDPI

Editorial

Nutritional Modulation of Dietary Sugars as a Strategy to Improve Insulin Resistance and Energy Balance in Diabetes

Paulo Matafome [1,2,3,4]

1 Polytechnic University of Coimbra, Coimbra Health School, 3046-854 Coimbra, Portugal; paulo.matafome@uc.pt
2 Coimbra Institute for Clinical and Biomedical Research (iCBR) and Institute of Physiology, Faculty of Medicine, University of Coimbra, 3000-548 Coimbra, Portugal
3 Center for Innovative Biomedicine and Biotechnology (CIBB), University of Coimbra, 3000-548 Coimbra, Portugal
4 Clinical Academic Center of Coimbra (CACC), 3000-548 Coimbra, Portugal

Lifestyle changes and less healthy behaviours include dietary changes toward increased consumption of Westernised diets and processed food. This is associated with the increasing prevalence of overweight in young adults and risk of obesity and associated pathologies later in life. The World Health Organization (WHO) established guidelines for free sugar intake in adults and children to be below 5–10% of total daily energy. However, recent studies support that it may actually be 15–20% in adults [1]. According to the National Portuguese Food and Physical Activity Survey report, the average national consumption of simple sugars (mono- and di-saccharides) is 90 g/day, contributing to an average of 19.8% for the total energy value and 17.3% in adults [2].

The consumption of added sugars contributes to an increased energy density in diet, leading to a positive energy balance, larger waist circumference, and weight gain, increasing the risk of obesity and type 2 diabetes [3,4]. Moreover, given the strong association between whole-body and abdominal fat mass with type 2 diabetes, cardiovascular diseases, and cancers, the guidelines of the World Health Organization (WHO) recommend 15–30% of total daily energy intake to be from fats and less than 10% intake of saturated fats. Fat accumulation and body mass index (BMI) were shown to be directly proportional to the excessive intake of energy in relation to expenditure, especially from foods rich in fats [5,6].

Sugars may be divided into two distinct groups: those naturally present and those added to foods. Natural or intrinsic sugars are naturally present in foods, such as fruit sugar (fructose), vegetables, honey, and sugars from dairy products (galactose and lactose). Added sugars are a large group of mono- and di-saccharides added to foods during processing, preparation, or at the table, with the objective of sweetening and increasing food palatability and shelf life, improving the texture, inhibiting the growth of microorganisms in high concentrations, provide functional structures, or increase accessibility. They are mostly found in sugary drinks, pastry products, cookies, fruit juices, energy drinks, nectars, fruit juices from concentrate, white bread, and breakfast cereals.

The impact of dietary sugars on the pathophysiological mechanisms of type 2 diabetes and its complications is not entirely understood. This Special Issue explores the association between the excessive consumption of dietary sugars, their sources and types, as well as their different impact on several features of type 2 diabetes aetiology and several physiological and pathophysiological processes and mechanisms of disease. In the articles published by Fernandes et al., Monteiro-Alfredo & Matafome, Garcia et al., and Mendes & Barra et al., the consumption and impact of dietary sugars on the gastrointestinal system is discussed. Fernandes et al. discuss the dietary sources of naturally occurring and added sugars, while Mendes & Barra et al. describe the role of different diets and dietary regimens in preventing post-prandial sugar increase and hyperinsulinemia. Moreover, Monteiro-Alfredo & Matafome and Garcia et al. explore the intestinal metabolism of dietary sugars, including

Citation: Matafome, P. Nutritional Modulation of Dietary Sugars as a Strategy to Improve Insulin Resistance and Energy Balance in Diabetes. *Diabetology* 2023, 4, 184–185. https://doi.org/10.3390/diabetology4020018

Received: 7 June 2023
Accepted: 7 June 2023
Published: 10 June 2023

the formation and absorption of advanced glycation end products and their impact on the gut microbiota. Regarding the impact of dietary sugars on other metabolic processes, Malta et al. describe the long-term alterations in beta-cell function caused by an increased and sustained consumption of sugars. Such consequences may include modifications of the mitochondrial function, generation of oxidative stress, and modulation of inflammatory pathways. These topics are covered by the reviews published by Diniz et al. and Barbosa & Carvalho. The impact of excessive and chronic sugar consumption may also arise from impaired energy balance and the development of addictive behaviors. The impact of sugars in the modulation of hypothalamic pathways is discussed by Capucho & Conde. Additionally, regarding the development of prevention strategies to avoid the negative impact of dietary sugars, Pedrosa et al. describe the role of exercise in reducing blood markers of glucose dysmetabolism. Importantly, the review published by Ferreira-Junior et al. demonstrates the importance of preventing excessive sugar consumption in critical phases of development since it may have long-term consequences.

Overall, this Special Issue covers an important topic with relevance not only from a scientific point-of-view but also from nutritional, policy, and industrial perspectives. We are currently subjected to increasing obesogenic pressures, with sugars being hidden in many foods, creating the perfect environment for the slow but consistent progression of metabolic dysfunction. This Special Issue aims to uncover the mechanisms involved and increase awareness of this escalating health problem.

Funding: This work was supported by the Portuguese Foundation of Science and Technology (Strategic Projects UIDB//04539/2020, UIDP//04539/ 2020, and LA/P/0058/2020: CIBB).

Conflicts of Interest: The authors declare no conflict of interest.

References

1. World Health Organization. *WHO Guideline: Sugars Intake for Adults and Children*; WHO Libr Cat Data; World Health Organization: Geneva, Switzerland, 2015.
2. Lopes, C.; Torres, D.; Oliveira, A.; Severo, M.; Alarcão, V.; Guiomar, S.; Mota, J.; Teixeira, P.; Ramos, E.; Rodrigues, S.; et al. *Inquérito Alimentar Nacional e de Atividade Fisica*; Direção-Geral Da Saúde: Lisbon, Portugal, 2017; Volume 14, p. 1341E.
3. Bes-Rastrollo, M.; Sayon-Orea, C.; Ruiz-Canela, M.; Martinez-Gonzalez, M.A. Impact of sugars and sugar taxation on body weight control: A comprehensive literature review. *Obesity* **2016**, *24*, 1410–1426. [CrossRef] [PubMed]
4. Pfinder, M.; Heise, T.L.; Boon, M.H.; Pega, F.; Fenton, C.; Griebler, U.; Gartlehner, G.; Sommer, I.; Katikireddi, S.V.; Lhachimi, S.K. Taxation of unprocessed sugar or sugar-added foods for reducing their consumption and preventing obesity or other adverse health outcomes. *Cochrane Database Syst. Rev.* **2020**, *2020*. [CrossRef] [PubMed]
5. Veum, V.L.; Laupsa-Borge, J.; Eng, Ø.; Rostrup, E.; Larsen, T.H.; Nordrehaug, J.E.; Nygård, O.K.; Sagen, J.V.; Gudbrandsen, O.A.; Dankel, S.N.; et al. Visceral adiposity and metabolic syndrome after very high-fat and low-fat isocaloric diets: A randomized controlled trial. *Am. J. Clin. Nutr.* **2017**, *105*, 85–99. [CrossRef] [PubMed]
6. Swainson, M.G.; Batterham, A.M.; Tsakirides, C.; Rutherford, Z.H.; Hind, K. Prediction of whole-body fat percentage and visceral adipose tissue mass from five anthropometric variables. *PLoS ONE* **2017**, *12*, e0177175. [CrossRef] [PubMed]

diabetology

MDPI

Review

Sources of Free and Added Sugars and Their Nutritional Impact in Diabetic Patients

Tatiana Fernandes [1], Ana Faria [2,*] and Helena Loureiro [2,*]

1 Centro Hospitalar e Universitário de Coimbra, Praceta Professor Mota Pinto, 3004-561 Coimbra, Portugal
2 Instituto Politécnico de Coimbra, Escola Superior de Tecnologia da Saúde de Coimbra, Rua 5 de Outubro—S. Martinho Bispo, 3046-854 Coimbra, Portugal
* Correspondence: ana.faria@estescoimbra.pt (A.F.); helenasoaresl@gmail.com (H.L.)

Abstract: A high consumption of sugar leads to an increase in caloric intake, which in turn will lead to a higher risk of developing health issues. Foods contain both naturally occurring sugars and added sugars. The World Health Organization recommends that the daily intake of free sugars be below 10% of the total daily energy intake. Food performs a key role in maintaining an adequate glycaemic control in people with diabetes. However, there is a low compliance to dietary recommendations, namely in the amount of sugar intake. This review article aims to assess and compare the intake of various types of sugars in the general population and among individuals with and without a diabetes diagnosis, identify the food sources that contribute to the intake of free and added sugars, and understand their impact on health. Studies performed on the general population found that the consumption of sugar was high, and that children and teens are more likely to exceed the recommended amounts. It was found that diabetics consume less total and added sugar than non-diabetics, as well as a less sugary drinks. Guidelines and public health policy measures aimed at limiting the intake of free and added sugars are needed in order to minimize the consumption of foods high in empty calories.

Keywords: sugar intake; free sugars; added sugars; diabetes

Citation: Fernandes, T.; Faria, A.; Loureiro, H. Sources of Free and Added Sugars and Their Nutritional Impact in Diabetic Patients. *Diabetology* **2022**, *3*, 634–638. https://doi.org/10.3390/diabetology3040049

Academic Editor: Peter Clifton

Received: 26 September 2022
Accepted: 7 December 2022
Published: 12 December 2022

1. Introduction

In recent years, sugar intake has become a public health concern due to its high consumption and connection to various health issues, such as obesity, cardiovascular diseases, diabetes, metabolic syndrome [1–4], tooth decay, nonalcoholic fatty liver disease, and some cancers [2].

Foods include several different types of sugars that can be naturally occurring or added to food.

Added sugars are sugars used in food processing and/or preparation, such as sucrose, brown sugar, corn syrup, dextrose, fructose, glucose, honey, molasses, inverted sugar, lactose, maltose, and fruit concentrates [5,6]. This kind of sugar excludes naturally occurring sugars in fruits, vegetables, whole-milk dairy products and juices, and/or fruit and vegetable purées.

The term 'free sugars' includes all added sugars and the naturally occurring sugars present in fruits and vegetables in the form of juices or purées. However, it excludes the sugars present in fruits, vegetables, and whole-milk dairy products.

All added sugars are free sugars, and both exclude the sugars naturally present in foods such as in fruits, vegetables, and whole-milk dairy, regardless of whether these are fresh, cooked, or dry [6,7].

Since free and added sugars have similar definitions, the World Health Organization (WHO) uses the term "free sugars" [1].

Total sugars are all the sugars presents in foods derived from any source [2,6].

Excess consumption of calories can lead to weight gain and consequently, obesity and its comorbidities. A high consumption of sugars, namely of added sugars, contributes to eating "empty" calories and, since they carry no nutrients, in excess they promote weight gain/obesity [1,3,8].

The types of sugar provided by different food sources present important differences in health risks. Eating excess calories, weight gain, diabetes, and tooth decay place free sugars as the primary cause of concern [6]. According to Mela et al. [6], these types of sugars should be the main focus of action in public health activities.

The WHO recommends a decrease in the consumption of free sugars to <10% of the total daily energy intake throughout life in children and adults, and, conditionally, also recommends an intake of <5% [1,6,9,10].

Diabetes is a challenging condition in terms of management and monitoring, as it requires important care by the patient, namely in regards to food. Nutritional therapy is key to an adequate glycaemic control [11–13]. However, studies show that there is a low compliance when it comes to dietary recommendations. According to Asaad et al. [12], eating above 10% of your daily total energy intake (DTEI) in sucrose increases blood sugar and triglycerides in people with type 2 diabetes.

This study aims to evaluate and compare the consumption of the various types of sugar (total, added, and free) in the general population and in people with or without a diabetes diagnosis, to identify food sources that contribute to eating free and added sugars, and to understand their effects on health.

2. Sources and Methods

Revision of the published literature between January of 2012 and April of 2022, on the consumption of total, free, and added sugars in people with or without a diabetes diagnosis. The electronic databases used were PubMed and Google Scholar, using a boolean operator (AND) and the keywords "free sugars", "added sugars", "diabetes", and "diabetic population".

The inclusion criteria of the selected articles are: intake of various types of sugars, individuals with and without diabetes, and identification of food sources that provide free and added sugars.

The selection of articles was considered by the date of publication (until 2012), title, abstract, and the full text.

3. Results and Discussion

In Europe, the energy intake derived from added sugars was 7.5% to 17%, and it was more significant in children and teens (11% to 17% of the DTEI) [2,14].

In Portugal, according to the 2015–2016 National Food and Physical Activity Survey, the national average intake of simple sugars was 84 g per day, making up 18.5% of the DTEI. As for the consumption of free sugars (7.5% of the DTEI), 24.3% of the Portuguese population exceeded the value recommended by the WHO, and a higher incidence was noted in children and teens. "Table" sugar added to food and beverages (21.4%), sweets (16.7%), and soft drinks (11.9%) were the food groups and subgroups that contributed most to the intake of free sugars [15].

A study performed in Switzerland on adults aged 18 to 75 years showed that the daily totalconsumption of added and free sugars accounted for 19%, 9%, and 11% of total energy intake, respectively. Sweets, drinks (soft drinks), and dairy products (yogurts) were the main food sources of added and free sugars. In younger adults (aged 18 to 29), most of these types of sugars came from soft drinks, while in older adults, sweet products such as honey, jams, cakes, and biscuits took up a more significant share [2].

In the Australian population, the intake of added sugars was found to be 10.8% of the total daily calorie intake. In regards to the WHO guidelines, more than half the sample had a higher intake of free sugars than recommended, and children and teens were more likely to exceed the recommended amount [16].

Between 2017 and 2018, 12.7% of the energy intake consumed by the United States population came from added sugars. This intake was greater in ages between 9 to 18 and lesser in the elderly (>71 years old). Irrespective of age, ethnicity, or income, sugary drinks and confectionery were the main food sources of added sugars in this population in 2011–2018 [10].

In Latin American countries, the intake of total sugars (20.1%) and added sugars (13.2%) was high. The 15–19 age range was that with the highest exhibited intake. Similarly to other studies, intake decreased with the increase in age [2,4,10].

A study conducted by Liu et al. [17], implemented in the Canadian population in 2015, showed similar results to previous studies. The average daily intake of total sugars was 105.6 g (21.6% of the DTEI), 57.1 g (11.1% of the DTEI) corresponded to added sugars, and 67.1 g (13.3% of the of the DTEI) to the consumption of free sugars. The food groups that most contributed to the intake of sugars in the diet of this population were desserts, sweets, and sugary drinks.

When assessing the consumption of sugars in individuals with diabetes, Wang et al.'s study [11] in the United States of America on Hispanic/Latino adults with and without a diabetes diagnosis, they found that people with diabetes ingested less total sugar (19.1% vs. 21.5% of total energy, $p = 0.002$) and less added sugar (9.8% vs. 12.1% of total energy, $p < 0.001$), as well as exhibiting a lower consumption of sugary drinks (8.8% vs. 11% of total energy, $p = 0.004$).

Asaad et al.'s study [12] assessed the intake of added sugar and the main food sources. According to the WHO guidelines, this sample reached the recommended added sugar intake (8.7 ± 4.8%), with desserts, yogurts, chocolates, breakfast cereal, and cakes being the main food sources of added sugars. The authors of this study found that individuals with diabetes consumed less total sugar compared to non-diabetics, probably because carbohydrates are the macronutrient with the highest impact on blood sugar.

As found by several studies, individuals diagnosed with diabetes have a greater degree of awareness when it comes to adopting healthy lifestyles and practicing healthy eating in order to obtain adequate glycaemic control [11,12,18].

A study conducted in Spain (in the year 2013) observed that diabetic adults consumed on average 24 g of added sugars per day, corresponding to 11% of their daily energy intake, while men and younger individuals (aged 18 to 44) had a greater intake of added sugars than this group. The food sources that contributed to the intake of such sugars were sugar, honey and syrups (19.4%), confectionery and baked goods (19.1%), and sweetened soft drinks (13.4%) [13]. A similar result was identified in a sample of subjects with type 1 diabetes, with an average age of 18, in which the intake of added sugars represented 12.4% of the total caloric intake, from sweetened drinks and sweets/desserts [19].

The majority of studies reported that sugary drinks are one of the food sources that most contributed to the intake of free and added sugars [2,8,10,11,15,19].

Research has identified a link between the intake of sugary drinks and between a higher risk of developing type 2 diabetes, with the added sugar content in drinks being the contributing factor to negative health outcomes [8,18]. Furthermore, individuals who consume this type of drinks have on average a more unhealthy lifestyle—less physical exercise, more tobacco consumption and calories, and a poor quality diet [20].

A study carried out with young people from Jordan identified a positive and significant relationship between body mass index and waist circumference in individuals who consumed drinks with added sugars. This relationship was justified by the high energy intake from these drinks, which resulted in a positive energy balance and increased adiposity [21].

Strategies such as reducing the consumption of these drinks prevents the occurrence of diabetes in the general population and allows for a greater control of this condition in individuals with type 2 diabetes, namely in terms of blood sugar levels, weight gain, and inflammation [22].

4. Conclusions

While nutrition aspects for patients with diabetes are defined [23], detailed nutritional evaluations and guidelines on the ill-effects of consuming free and added sugars still remain unexplored.

Guidelines and public health policy measures aimed at limiting the intake of free and added sugars are needed [14], such as an overhaul of added-sugar products (soft drinks, yogurts, dairy desserts, confectionery products) particularly in the amount of sugar, which should be reduced and regulated [2,14], a reduction of serving sizes, a taxation of sugary drinks [2,15], and a clear messaging on minimizing the consumption of foods high in empty calories and in promoting healthy drinks and foods [16].

In regards to food labeling, it is essential that it is suitable and that it clearly identifies free and added sugars in food products [1].

The increased prevalence of diabetes and prediabetes associated with an increase in obesity indicates the need for effective strategies that promote the adoption of healthy eating habits and alternatives to a high intake of free sugars [3].

Author Contributions: Conceptualization, T.F., A.F. and H.L.; formal analysis, T.F. and H.L; investigation, T.F. and H.L.; data curation, T.F.; writing—original draft preparation, T.F.; writing—review and editing, T.F.; visualization, T.F., A.F. and H.L. All authors have read and agreed to the published version of the manuscript.

Funding: This research received no external funding.

Institutional Review Board Statement: Not applicable.

Informed Consent Statement: Not applicable.

Data Availability Statement: The data presented in this study are available on request from the corresponding author.

Conflicts of Interest: The authors declare no conflict of interest.

References

1. Ruiz, E.; Rodriguez, P.; Valero, T.; Ávila, J.M.; Aranceta-Bartrina, J.; Gil, Á.; González-Gross, M.; Ortega, R.M.; Serra-Majem, L.; Varela-Moreiras, G. Dietary Intake of Individual (Free and Intrinsic) Sugars and Food Sources in the Spanish Population: Findings from the ANIBES Study. *Nutrients* **2017**, *9*, 275. [CrossRef] [PubMed]
2. Chatelan, A.; Gaillard, P.; Kruseman, M.; Keller, A. Total, Added, and Free Sugar Consumption and Adherence to Guidelines in Switzerland: Results from the First National Nutrition Survey MenuCH. *Nutrients* **2019**, *11*, 1117. [CrossRef] [PubMed]
3. Warshaw, H.; Edelman, S.V. Practical Strategies to Help Reduce Added Sugars Consumption to Support Glycemic and Weight Management Goals. *Clin. Diabetes* **2021**, *39*, 45–56. [CrossRef] [PubMed]
4. Fisberg, M.; Kovalskys, I.; Gómez, G.; Rigotti, A.; Sanabria, L.Y.C.; García, M.C.Y.; Torres, R.G.P.; Herrera-Cuenca, M.; Zimberg, I.Z.; Koletzko, B.; et al. Total and Added Sugar Intake: Assessment in Eight Latin American Countries. *Nutrients* **2018**, *10*, 389. [CrossRef] [PubMed]
5. Pfinder, M.; Katikireddi, S.V.; Pega, F.; Gartlehner, G.; Fenton, C.; Griebler, U.; Sommer, I.; Heise, T.L.; Lhachimi, S.K. Taxation of Unprocessed Sugar or Sugar-Added Foods for Reducing Their Consumption and Preventing Obesity or Other Adverse Health Outcomes. *Cochrane Database Syst. Rev.* **2016**. [CrossRef]
6. Mela, D.J.; Woolner, E.M. Perspective: Total, Added, or Free? What Kind of Sugars Should We Be Talking About? *Adv. Nutr.* **2018**, *9*, 63–69. [CrossRef]
7. Sluik, D.; van Lee, L.; Engelen, A.I.; Feskens, E.J.M. Total, Free, and Added Sugar Consumption and Adherence to Guidelines: The Dutch National Food Consumption Survey 2007–2010. *Nutrients* **2016**, *8*, 70. [CrossRef]
8. Veit, M.; van Asten, R.; Olie, A.; Prinz, P. The Role of Dietary Sugars, Overweight, and Obesity in Type 2 Diabetes Mellitus: A Narrative Review. *Eur. J. Clin. Nutr.* **2022**, *76*, 1497–1501. [CrossRef]
9. Guidelines Review Committee, Nutrition and Food Safety, WHO South-East Asia. *Guideline: Sugars Intake for Adults and Children*; World Health Organization: Geneva, Switzerland, 2015; Volume 57, pp. 1716–1722.
10. Ricciuto, L.; Fulgoni, V.L.; Gaine, P.C.; Scott, M.O.; DiFrancesco, L. Sources of Added Sugars Intake Among the U.S. Population: Analysis by Selected Sociodemographic Factors Using the National Health and Nutrition Examination Survey 2011–18. *Front. Nutr.* **2021**, *8*, 687643. [CrossRef]
11. Wang, X.; Jung, M.; Mossavar-Rahmani, Y.; Sotres-Alvarez, D.; Espinoza Giacinto, R.A.; Pirzada, A.; Reina, S.A.; Casagrande, S.S.; Wang, T.; Avilés-Santa, M.L.; et al. Macronutrient Intake, Diagnosis Status, and Glycemic Control among US Hispanics/Latinos with Diabetes. *J. Clin. Endocrinol. Metab.* **2016**, *101*, 1856–1864. [CrossRef]
12. Asaad, G.; Chan, C.B. Food Sources of Sodium, Saturated Fat, and Added Sugar in the Physical Activity and Nutrition for Diabetes in Alberta (PANDA) Trial. *Appl. Physiol. Nutr. Metab.* **2017**, *42*, 1270–1276. [CrossRef] [PubMed]
13. Guallar-Castillón, P.; Muñoz-Pareja, M.; Aguilera, M.T.; León-Muñoz, L.M.; Rodríguez-Artalejo, F. Food Sources of Sodium, Saturated Fat and Added Sugar in the Spanish Hypertensive and Diabetic Population. *Atherosclerosis* **2013**, *229*, 198–205. [CrossRef]

14. Azaïs-Braesco, V.; Sluik, D.; Maillot, M.; Kok, F.; Moreno, L.A. A Review of Total & Added Sugar Intakes and Dietary Sources in Europe. *Nutr. J.* **2017**, *16*, 6. [CrossRef] [PubMed]
15. Lopes, C.; Torres, D.; Oliveira, A.; Severo, M.; Alarcão, V.; Guiomar, S.; Mota, J.; Teixeira, P.; Rodrigues, S.; Lobato, L.; et al. *Inquérito Alimentar Nacional e de Atividade Física-IAN-AF, 2015–2016*; Universidade do Porto: Porto, Portugal, 2017; Volume 112.
16. Lei, L.; Rangan, A.; Flood, V.M.; Louie, J.C.Y. Dietary Intake and Food Sources of Added Sugar in the Australian Population. *Br. J. Nutr.* **2016**, *115*, 868–877. [CrossRef] [PubMed]
17. Liu, S.; Munasinghe, L.L.; Ohinmaa, A.; Veugelers, P.J. Added, Free and Total Sugar Content and Consumption of Foods and Beverages in Canada. *Health Rep.* **2020**, *31*, 14–24. [CrossRef] [PubMed]
18. Xu, F.; Park, S.; Siegel, K.R. Factors Associated With Frequency of Sugar-Sweetened Beverage Consumption Among US Adults With Diabetes or Prediabetes. *Am. J. Health Promot.* **2017**, *32*, 1489–1497. [CrossRef] [PubMed]
19. The, N.S.; Couch, S.C.; Urbina, E.M.; Crandell, J.L.; Liese, A.D.; Dabelea, D.; Kim, G.J.; Tooze, J.A.; Lawrence, J.M.; Mayer-Davis, E.J. Body Mass Index Z-Score Modifies the Association between Added Sugar Intake and Arterial Stiffness in Youth with Type 1 Diabetes: The Search Nutrition Ancillary Study. *Nutrients* **2019**, *11*, 1752. [CrossRef]
20. Khan, T.A.; Sievenpiper, J.L. Controversies about Sugars: Results from Systematic Reviews and Meta-Analyses on Obesity, Cardiometabolic Disease and Diabetes. *Eur. J. Nutr.* **2016**, *55*, 25–43. [CrossRef]
21. Bawadi, H.; Khataybeh, T.; Obeidat, B.; Kerkadi, A.; Tayyem, R.; Banks, A.D.; Subih, H. Sugar-Sweetened Beverages Contribute Significantly to College Students' Daily Caloric Intake in Jordan: Soft Drinks Are Not the Major Contributor. *Nutrients* **2019**, *11*, 1058. [CrossRef]
22. Tseng, T.-S.; Lin, W.-T.; Gonzalez, G.V.; Kao, Y.-H.; Chen, L.-S.; Lin, H.-Y. Sugar Intake from Sweetened Beverages and Diabetes: A Narrative Review. *World J. Diabetes* **2021**, *12*, 1530–1538. [CrossRef]
23. Narayanan, S.; Bhutiani, N.; Adamson, D.T.; Jones, C.M. Pancreatectomy, Islet Cell Transplantation, and Nutrition Considerations. *Nutr. Clin. Pract.* **2021**, *36*, 385–397. [CrossRef] [PubMed]

diabetology

Review

Diet Modifications towards Restoration of Insulin Sensitivity and Daily Insulin Fluctuations in Diabetes

Ana Magalhães [1,†], Cátia Barra [1,2,*,†], Ana Borges [1,3] and Lèlita Santos [1,2,4]

1 Internal Medicine Service, Coimbra Hospital and University Centre, 3000-548 Coimbra, Portugal
2 Coimbra Institute of Clinical and Biomedical Research (iCBR), Faculty of Medicine and Center of Innovative Biomedicine and Biotechnology (CIBB), University of Coimbra, 3000-548 Coimbra, Portugal
3 Faculty of Medicine, University of Coimbra, 3000-548 Coimbra, Portugal
4 CIMAGO Research Centre, Faculty of Medicine, University of Coimbra, 3000-548 Coimbra, Portugal
* Correspondence: 12071@chuc.min-saude.pt
† These authors contributed equally to this work.

Abstract: The circadian rhythm is essential in order to maintain metabolic homeostasis and insulin sensitivity. Disruption of circadian mechanisms is associated with the development of metabolic diseases, such as diabetes. Lifestyle changes such as an equilibrated diet and physical activity are known to improve glycaemic control in diabetic patients. One of the mechanisms possibly involved in such an improvement is the restoration of insulin circadian rhythms. There are several available dietary schemes based on circadian rhythms. Some of them are associated with better regulation of daily insulin fluctuations and the improvement of Type 2 Diabetes and metabolic syndrome. In the current review, we aim to explore how the different types of diet can impact glucose metabolism and insulin sensitivity in patients with diabetes, highlighting the interactions with the mechanisms of circadian insulin rhythm and the prevention of hyperinsulinemia.

Keywords: daily insulin fluctuation; insulin sensitivity; diets; circadian rhythm

Citation: Magalhães, A.; Barra, C.; Borges, A.; Santos, L. Diet Modifications towards Restoration of Insulin Sensitivity and Daily Insulin Fluctuations in Diabetes. *Diabetology* **2022**, *3*, 606–614. https://doi.org/10.3390/diabetology3040046

Academic Editor: Peter Clifton

Received: 30 September 2022
Accepted: 18 November 2022
Published: 22 November 2022

Publisher's Note: MDPI stays neutral with regard to jurisdictional claims in published maps and institutional affiliations.

1. Introduction

Insulin was discovered by Frederick Banting and Charles Best in 1921. It is a pancreatic beta-cell anabolic hormone initially produced by as pre-insulin and then as proinsulin after a maturation process [1]. Subsequently, it is translocated from the endoplasmic reticulum to the Golgi apparatus, where it is cleaved into C-peptide and insulin, which are simultaneously released by exocytosis [2]. Its production by pancreatic beta cells is enhanced in response to glucose, and it is responsible for maintaining constant blood levels of glucose and metabolic homeostasis. However, it has been demonstrated that amino acids and fatty acids are also capable of stimulating insulin secretion [3,4]. Its secretion from pancreatic beta cells is biphasic: the first phase occurs with a rapid release, while the second phase is characterized by a more sustained and less elevated release [5]. Insulin levels are increased in the postprandial period when the circulating glucose levels increase, making the first phase very significant. In this phase, insulin inhibits glucagon secretion from the pancreatic alpha cells through paracrine action at the beginning of the meal. On the other hand, the second phase is critical for maintaining this inhibition and increasing glucose storage and utilization [6]. Thirty minutes after the beginning of the meal, insulin suppresses lipolysis in the adipose tissue by inactivating the hormone-sensitive lipase, leading to a decrease in non-esterified fatty acids (NEFA) and glycerol in the blood [7,8]. The lower blood NEFA and higher insulin levels induce the suppression of glucose production in the liver and an increase in glucose utilization (glycolysis) by the muscle [3,9,10]. Insulin and glucagon secretion, as well as glucose homeostasis, are also regulated by the incretins, which are secreted by the gut in response to food intake [11,12]. Glucagon-like peptide-1 (GLP-1) and glucose-dependent insulinotropic polypeptide (GIP) are the two major incretins derived from gut neuroendocrine cells and are involved in these mechanisms, and their receptors may be found both in alpha and beta cells [11,13].

Insulin secretion dysregulation due to several causes promotes the development of diabetes. Type 1 diabetes (T1D) is characterized by auto-immune destruction of beta cells, while type 2 diabetes (T2D) is related to the development of insulin resistance, which is associated with obesity and metabolic syndrome. In T2D, beta-cell destruction is also observed through their progressive exhaustion and dysfunction in a later phase [14,15]. Consequently, beta-cell hyperplasia and a hyperinsulinemic state are often observed in obese patients in order to compensate for chronic low-grade inflammation and insulin resistance [14,16,17]. Moreover, hyperinsulinemia itself contributes to insulin resistance due to insulin receptor downregulation [11]. Lifestyle changes such as an equilibrated diet and physical exercise may prevent these events and thus contribute to maintaining a normal weight and insulin sensitivity in the peripheral tissues.

2. Circadian Rhythm Influences Insulin Secretion

The circadian rhythm is essential for maintaining a normal body physiology. It is mediated by specific components that are controlled by the daily light–dark and feeding–fasting cycles. The central nervous system plays an important role in the circadian rhythm through synapse networking, which acts in different brain regions and in endocrine cells, contributing to the circadian regulation of metabolism [18]. These outputs are integrated into the hypothalamus, which is responsible for hunger–satiety, thermoregulation, sleep–arousal, and osmolarity [19].

The metabolic activity of several organs is also mediated by their internal clocks and circadian rhythms. In the intestine, the expression of sodium-glucose transport protein 1 (SGLT-1) has a rhythmic cycle, which is increased when the glucose intake is anticipated. Similar mechanisms regulate insulin secretion. Besides being regulated by glucose levels and incretins, its exocytosis also has a circadian regulation, possibly because incretins also have a circadian rhythm themselves [20]. Some studies in healthy human subjects have shown daily fluctuations in glucose tolerance, suggesting that it is greatest in the morning, while a significant decrease occurs during the night [21,22]. This is not only because of the oscillations in peripheral insulin sensitivity, but also the variations of glucose-stimulated insulin secretion during the daily 24 h period [23].

Uncoupling protein 2 (UCP2) has been described to influence metabolism, as it is expressed by endogenous circadian oscillators in pancreatic islets and acts in beta cells as a negative regulator of glucose-stimulated insulin secretion (GSIS). As mentioned before, insulin regulates the metabolic response to fasting and its suppression is crucial to allow for endogenous glucose production in the liver and lipolysis in the adipose tissue in order to release metabolic fuel. Therefore, Ucp2/UCP2 has been suggested to coordinate insulin secretion according to nutrient ingestion, so an upregulation of Ucp2/UCP2 prevents hypoglycaemia during the fasting period by inhibiting insulin secretion and promoting fuel mobilization [24,25]. This type of regulation influences the activity of several other endocrine pathways such as melatonin, glucocorticoids, and growth hormone (GH) [20]. GH and cortisol secretion are regulated by their own circadian rhythm, and are higher in the nocturnal period, which contributes to insulin resistance in the early morning hours [22].

It has been demonstrated that chronic disruption of these circadian mechanisms is related to the development of metabolic diseases, as established by several studies in shift workers [26,27]. In a retrospective study conducted by Garaulet and her collaborators, eating early (lunch time before 15:00 p.m.) results in enhanced weight loss effectiveness, suggesting a relation between eating intervals and the day–night cycle in the metabolism [28]. Other studies have revealed that time-restricted feeding is capable of improving metabolic diseases due to sustained diurnal rhythms and imposing daily feeding–fasting cycles [29,30]. Similar to what happens with GH and cortisol, melatonin (Figure 1) also promotes a hyperglycaemic state in the evening, given that melatonin binding to its receptor in pancreatic islets inhibits insulin release from the beta cells [31]. Reciprocal interactions between metabolism and the circadian clock imply that nutrition quality, quantity, and daily eating patterns can affect diurnal rhythms, which in turn determine whole-body physiology.

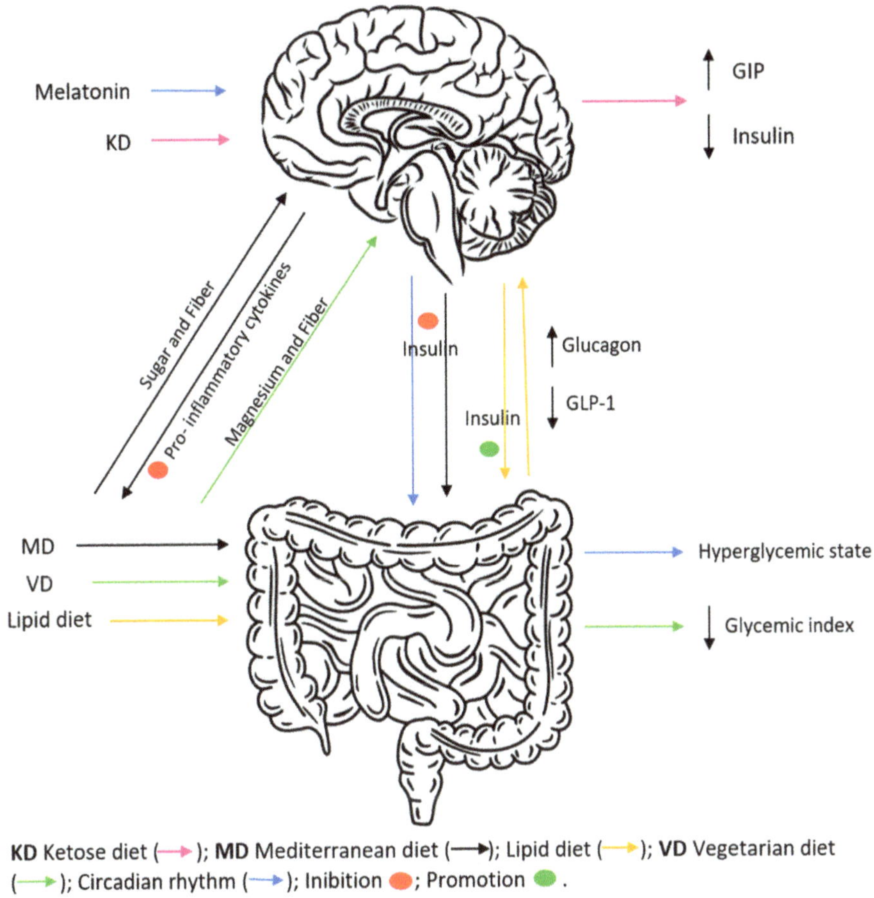

Figure 1. Effects of different diets on insulin and incretins secretion, as well as hyperglycaemic and inflammatory states. KD, characterized by the ingestion of <50 g of carbohydrates/day, promotes a decrease in insulin and increase in glucagon and GIP fasting levels. MD, because of its higher fiber supply and reduced sugar ingestion, is capable of decreasing blood insulin levels and increasing GIP secretion, similarly decreasing pro-inflammatory cytokine activation and reducing the risk of diabetes development. VD, based on reduced calorie ingestion and being rich in magnesium and fibre, promotes a decrease in GI. A lipid diet is associated with diabetes development by increasing glucagon secretion and decreasing GLP-1.

3. The Impact of Different Diets on the Levels of Insulin Secretion

3.1. The Impact of Diet

Nowadays, most diets that are called healthy can be included in a few categories: they match the Mediterranean Diet, or they are low in fat, low in carbohydrates (CH), or are vegetarian [32]. Nutrition is considered one of the pillars for the prevention and treatment of several diseases, namely metabolic syndrome [33]. Besides the amount of food ingested, growing attention has been devoted to the quality of macronutrients and the role they play in the regulation of T2D [34,35]. The current discussion about food standards suggests that it is not just a question of quantity, but also of quality and, importantly, time and schedule. For example, eating most calories and carbs at lunchtime or in the early afternoon, avoiding late dinners, and keeping the number of meals and the timing of meals consistent, all play a role in regulating postprandial blood glucose and insulin sensitivity [36].

This section of the review will focus on postprandial insulin, and the long-term insulin response in relation to the glycaemic index (GI), the area under the curve (AUC) of the glucose response after CH consumption [37].

3.2. Mediterranean Diet

The Mediterranean Diet emerged in the 1960s as the diet with the most beneficial impact on health and the one recommended by experts. This diet is characterized mainly by the consumption of vegetables, with the regular consumption of protein (meat, fish, or egg), CH, and a limited amount of fats, usually from olive oil. Nonetheless, it is a diet low in fat and rich in vitamins with antioxidant and anti-inflammatory properties [35]. Therefore, as it decreases the activation of the pro-inflammatory cytokines (Figure 1), it also reduces chronic inflammation and the risk of T2D. As it includes a low consumption of sugar/CH, it also has a role in regulating diabetes. So, it is suggested that by resulting in a greater supply of fibre and less sugar, it is effective at decreasing the load of this component on the body, while also decreasing the circulating insulin levels [38].

3.3. Vegetarian Diet

Adherence to a vegetarian diet is growing worldwide. This is characterized by the exclusion of foods of an animal origin. However, if this diet is not supplemented, macro and micronutrient deficiencies such as omega-3 fatty acids, iron, vitamin D, calcium, zinc, iodine, and vitamin B12 may occur [32]. The reinforced intake of vegetables and cereals reduces the risk of T2D as they are rich in magnesium and fibre (Figure 1). The insulin signalling pathway is magnesium-dependent and fibre helps to lower the GI [39]. The low GI of this diet may explain the lower cardiovascular risk and greater insulin sensitivity compared with omnivores [37].

Within the scope of T2D, a plant-based diet will reduce body weight, as it reduces the ingested calories, and increases postprandial metabolism [34]. Some studies suggest that vegetarians have a lower amount of intramuscular lipids than omnivores, and this proportion also occurs at a hepatic level. By having this metabolic (catabolism) effect, it will decrease HbA1c and postprandial lipids. Visceral fat reduction also decreases the levels of plasma inflammatory adipokines and oxidative stress markers, which may have an effect on beta cell function and insulin regulation. An unexpected effect of this diet is that it increases the thermic effect of food, supporting this theory of catabolism [40]. The question that arises in this diet is its suitability for the entire population as it is a difficult diet to maintain, at least for the Western population, as a high intake of CH has to be monitored by a nutritionist [32].

3.4. Paleolithic Diet

This diet is based on the consumption of fruits, vegetables, eggs, fish, and meat, with the latter as a source of protein. Thus, it excludes all processed food, including dairy products. Thus, it contains less CH but a greater protein intake [41]. In fact, the distribution of nutrients occurs as follows: 35% lipids, 35% CH, and 30% protein [42]. The Paleolithic diet causes a reduction in insulin concentration after a meal, that is, less insulin is needed with this nutrient distribution than with other diets [43]. Studies have suggested that this approach decreases insulin secretion in the long-term and increases beta cell sensitivity to postprandial glucose load [42]. However, Genoni et al. suggest that this adaptation may not be beneficial in terms of intestinal motility [44]. Biologically, a catabolic state is stimulated and postprandial glucagon suppression is observed. Together with insulin secretion, this may result from improved postprandial secretion of the incretins GLP-1 and GIP into circulation. Their increase also promotes satiety and thus weight loss [41].

4. Diets That Promote Ketosis

This group of diets is divided into three types: low in CH, normoprotein, and high in lipids, such as the ketogenic diet. It also includes the famous «fasting» and calorie restriction, which increase ketosis due to the lack of calories. Despite a restriction of nutrients, some studies have considered this type of diet more healthy as it helps to preserve muscle mass, increase weight loss, reduce appetite, and above all decrease insulin resistance and circulating insulin levels [45,46].

4.1. Ketogenic Diet

It consists of a normocaloric diet well known for rapid weight loss. However, in terms of insulin patterns and its effect on the liver, it is still controversial [47]. The proposal is to ingest less than 50 g of CH per day, which will mimic a catabolic state. Insulin secretion will decrease as the main nutrient will be ketone bodies (from lipids) as an alternative substrate [45]. Fasting glucagon and GIP levels increase, while, after ingestion, postprandial glucose and insulin AUC are lower than in a control meal (Figure 1). The increased adiponectin observed after this diet may also promote insulin sensitivity [46].

4.2. Lipid-Modified Diet

As would be expected, this diet may increase the risk of obesity and insulin resistance [48], but some studies claim it is a matter of quantity. The type of ingested lipids affects the insulin signalling cascade. Contrary to expectations, intervention studies have reported that replacing monounsaturated with saturated lipids alters the plasma fatty acids, but may increase insulin sensitivity [34]. However, some studies report that this diet causes insulin resistance. A 2-week lipid-rich diet leads to insulin resistance in muscle tissue due to metabolic changes, specifically in the mitochondria (incomplete oxidation of molecules), and impaired signalling of the insulin cascade [49]. Given that this type of diet causes obesity, this may have other consequences, such as a decreased secretion of GLP-1 (Figure 1) [41]. Thus, the ratio between insulin and glucagon production in the pancreas is changed, leading to an increased appetite and increased caloric intake, which will cause an overstimulation of insulin and induce resistance [41].

4.3. Low Carb Diet (LCD)

This diet is often used by nutritionists as it promotes weight loss in a short period of time and, consequently, an improvement in the glycaemic profile. This diet is based on the consumption of vegetables and protein, removing virtually all CH (consuming < 130 g/day, the main foods originating glucose) [50]. In this context, the mathematical formula is simple: reducing the intake of glucose (present in CH) reduces hyperinsulinemia, which can be adapted for patients with diabetes [51]. There is evidence that this diet allows 93% of patients to regress to pre-diabetes, 46% of patients no longer need medication, and 60% of patients regress from diabetes within 1 year [51]. However, it has to be noted that a low glycaemic diet (GD) is not a low GI diet [52]. LCD improves the glycaemic profile because it rapidly increases postprandial insulin levels. However, a high glycaemic peak will cause patients to have less satiety and avoid a further increase in dietary intake [46].

4.4. Diet Rich in Carbohydrates

Controversial studies report that the ingestion of a diet rich in CH and fibre can lead to normoglycemia in prediabetic individuals [53]. After eating a meal, insulin in fat cells stimulates the entry of glucose into the tissues, decreasing the release of lipids and inhibiting the production of ketone bodies. Thus, this diet will produce hyperinsulinemia that will force the deposition of lipids instead of their oxidation [54]. The mechanisms are not clear; there are studies reporting that a diet rich in CH reduces blood glucose through glucose metabolism at the muscle level, improving the glycaemic profile in the short and long term [55]. This occurs if CH is not refined, with an increased adiponectin concentration, a decrease in body weight, and thus an improvement in the metabolic profile [56]. However, it is not clear what would be the long-term effects on beta cell function, because their overstimulation is expected to increase the risk of exhaustion.

Once again, nutrients are paramount, and diets with a GI < 55 are digested slowly and those with a high GI (>70) are digested quickly [52]. Importantly, high GI foods can alter leptin by interfering with satiety beyond the absorption spectrum [57]. So, foods that contain CH, such as vegetables and fruit, have better GI values, satisfying appetite for a longer time and improving the glycaemic profile [52].

4.5. Caloric Restriction

This dietary intervention consists of reducing the caloric intake by 25–30% from the baseline, but without restricting the necessary nutrients, that is, decreasing the quantity without decreasing the quality [45]. This diet can exacerbate some metabolic problems as it can increase appetite and stress hormones [54]. In this catabolic context, glucagon is favored and the secretion of GLP-1 is inhibited [41]. As a consequence, the hepatic glucose output is increased. However, pancreatic apoptosis decreases and insulin sensitivity increases, mainly due to the lower insulinemia [45]. It is especially problematic in patients with T2D, possibly causing hypoglycaemia and difficulties in the long-term regulation of glucose metabolism. Caloric restriction is more suitable for patients in the early stages of metabolic dysregulation, where it will favour body weight and fat mass loss, while decreasing lipotoxicity in the muscle, liver, and adipose tissue. This will decrease low-grade inflammation and increase insulin sensitivity. Thus, caloric restriction is suitable to prevent insulin resistance and beta-cell exhaustion in patients with obesity or prediabetes, although it is a dietary scheme that is very hard to follow by patients with T2D (reviewed by Joaquim et al., 2022 [58]). For patients with T2D, other less severe schemes are recommended, such as time-restricting fasting (TRF). In this dietary approach, patients are recommended to eat only during one part of the day, not consuming any calories during the other part, usually for at least 10 h. This approach often does not require caloric restriction, only fasting for half of the day in order to regulate relevant biological mechanisms such as circadian rhythms, stress hormones suppression, and autophagy (reviewed by Joaquim et al., 2022 [58]). As mentioned above, dietary consumption at specific times may coordinate the response to the presence or absence of nutrients, namely their gut metabolization and absorption; insulin secretion and action; and all the necessary changes in the liver, muscle, and adipose tissue metabolism. TRF has been shown to promote overnight mobilization of energy reserves through lipolysis, lipogenesis, and hepatic glucose production, contributing to a higher catabolic activity [59–61]. The rhythmic regulation of SGLT1 in the gut and UCP2 in beta cells, as already discussed, may in fact explain the positive effects of this type of diet on the beta-cell function and insulin sensitivity. It is possible that the overnight suppression of insulin may be a key factor in better diurnal insulin sensitivity and preserved beta-cell function (reviewed by Joaquim et al., 2022 [58]).

5. Conclusions

In this review, we focus on daily insulin fluctuation and glucose metabolism, as well as the influence of diet on these mechanisms. Metabolic homeostasis is highly coordinated by the circadian rhythm, which regulates insulin and glucagon secretion in order to maintain a normal fuel balance between tissues. However, it is well known that disruption of these mechanisms can lead to metabolic disease development, such as T2D. Current dietary habits are known to cause beta-cell overstimulation due to the high consumption of CH, especially refined ones. This will not only cause long-term beta-cell exhaustion but also insulin resistance, as hyperinsulinemia is one of the major drivers of insulin receptor inactivation. Nowadays, there are several diets known to improve insulin sensitivity and better control glycaemic profile in patients with T2D. Postprandial hyperglycaemia depends mainly on meal composition, but other factors also contribute to its magnitude, such as glucose absorption; secretion; and the action of incretin hormones, insulin, and glucagon. Thus, it is important to evaluate the quality of the nutrients rather than only their quantity, and, most importantly, their glycaemic impact. In T2D, it is important to adjust the diet to control glycemia after meals and the postprandial and fasting insulin levels.

Author Contributions: Conceptualization: A.M., C.B., A.B. and L.S. Methodology: A.M. and C.B.; A.B. and L.S. Writing—original draft preparation: A.M. and C.B. Writing-review and editing: A.B. and L.S.; Supervision: A.B. and L.S. All authors have read and agreed to the published version of the manuscript.

Funding: This work was supported by Foundation for Science and Technology (FCT), Portugal (Pest UID/NEU/04539/2013 and UID/NEU/04539/2019: CNC.IBILI; Pest UIDB/04539/2020 and UIDP/04539/2020: CIBB).

Institutional Review Board Statement: Not applicable.

Informed Consent Statement: Not applicable.

Data Availability Statement: The data presented in this study are available on request from the corresponding author.

Acknowledgments: Cátia Barra is a CIBB member, who is supported by the Portuguese Science and Technology Foundation (FCT), Strategic Projects UIDB/04539/2020 and UIDBP/4539/2020.

Conflicts of Interest: The authors declare no conflict of interest.

References

1. Bunney, P.E.; Zink, A.N.; Holm, A.A.; Billington, C.J.; Kotz, C.M. Orexin activation counteracts decreases in nonexercise activity thermogenesis (NEAT) caused by high-fat diet. *Physiol. Behav.* **2017**, *176*, 139–148. [CrossRef]
2. Fu, Z.; Gilbert, E.R.; Liu, D. Regulation of Insulin Synthesis and Secretion and Pancreatic Beta-Cell Dysfunction in Diabetes. *Curr. Diabetes Rev.* **2012**, *9*, 25–53. [CrossRef]
3. Dimitriadis, G.D.; Maratou, E.; Kountouri, A.; Board, M.; Lambadiari, V. Regulation of postabsorptive and postprandial glucose metabolism by insulin-dependent and insulin-independent mechanisms: An integrative approach. *Nutrients* **2021**, *13*, 159. [CrossRef]
4. Newsholme, P.; Cruzat, V.; Arfuso, F.; Keane, K. Nutrient regulation of insulin secretion and action. *J. Endocrinol.* **2014**, *221*, R105–R120. [CrossRef]
5. Seino, S.; Shibasaki, T.; Minami, K. Dynamics of insulin secretion in obesity. *J. Clin. Investig.* **2011**, *121*, 2118–2125. [CrossRef]
6. Steiner, K.E.; Mouton, S.M.; Bowles, C.R.; Williams, P.E.; Cherrington, A.D. The relative importance of first- and second-phase insulin secretion in countering the action of glucagon on glucose turnover in the conscious dog. *Diabetes* **1982**, *31*, 964–972. [CrossRef]
7. Miles, J.M.; Wooldridge, D.; Grellner, W.J.; Windsor, S.; Isley, W.L.; Klein, S.; Harris, W.S. Nocturnal and postprandial free fatty acid kinetics in normal and type 2 diabetic subjects: Effects of insulin sensitization therapy. *Diabetes* **2003**, *52*, 675–681. [CrossRef]
8. Dimitriadis, G.; Boutati, E.; Lambadiari, V.; Mitrou, P.; Maratou, E.; Brunel, P.; Raptis, S.A. Restoration of early insulin secretion after a meal in type 2 diabetes: Effects on lipid and glucose metabolism. *Eur. J. Clin. Investig.* **2004**, *34*, 490–497. [CrossRef]
9. Ferrannini, E.; Barrett, E.J.; Bevilacqua, S.; DeFronzo, R.A. Effect of fatty acids on glucose production and utilization in man. *J. Clin. Investig.* **1983**, *72*, 1737–1747. [CrossRef]
10. Groop, L.C.; Bonadonna, R.C.; DelPrato, S.; Ratheiser, K.; Zyck, K.; Ferrannini, E.; DeFronzo, R.A. Glucose and free fatty acid metabolism in non-insulin-dependent diabetes mellitus. Evidence for multiple sites of insulin resistance. *J. Clin. Investig.* **1989**, *84*, 205–213. [CrossRef]
11. Boer, G.A.; Holst, J.J. Increatin Hormones and Type 2 Diabetes Mellitus—Mechanistic Insights and Therapeutic Approches. *Biology* **2020**, *9*, 473. [CrossRef]
12. Nauck, M.A.; Meier, J.J. Incretin hormones: Their role in health and disease. *Diabetes Obes. Metab.* **2018**, *20*, 5–21. [CrossRef]
13. Heller, R.S.; Kieffer, T.J.; Habener, J.F. Insulinotropic glucagon-like peptide I receptor expression in glucagon- producing α-cells of the rat endocrine pancreas. *Diabetes* **1997**, *46*, 785–791. [CrossRef]
14. Christensen, A.A.; Gannon, M. The Beta Cell in Type 2 Diabetes. *Curr. Diab. Rep.* **2019**, *19*, 81. [CrossRef]
15. Halban, P.A.; Polonsky, K.S.; Bowden, D.W.; Hawkins, M.A.; Ling, C.; Mather, K.J.; Powers, A.C.; Rhodes, C.J.; Sussel, L.; Weir, G.C. β-Cell failure in type 2 diabetes: Postulated mechanisms and prospects for prevention and treatment. *Diabetes Care* **2014**, *37*, 1751–1758. [CrossRef]
16. Murai, N.; Saito, N.; Kodama, E.; Iida, T.; Mikura, K.; Imai, H.; Kaji, M.; Hashizume, M.; Kigawa, Y.; Koizumi, G.; et al. Insulin and Proinsulin Dynamics Progressively Deteriorate from within the Normal Range Toward Impaired Glucose Tolerance. *J. Endocr. Soc.* **2020**, *4*, bvaa066. [CrossRef]
17. Quan, W.; Jo, E.K.; Lee, M.S. Role of pancreatic β-cell death and inflammation in diabetes. *Diabetes Obes. Metab.* **2013**, *15*, 141–151. [CrossRef]
18. Mohawk, J.A.; Green, C.B.; Takahashi, J.S. Central and Peripheral clocks. *Annu. Rev. Neurosci.* **2012**, *35*, 445–462. [CrossRef]

19. Panda, S. Circadian physiology of metabolism. *Physiol. Behav.* **2016**, *176*, 139–148. [CrossRef]
20. Perelis, M.; Marcheva, B.; Moynihan Ramsey, K.; Schipma, M.J.; Hutchison, A.L.; Taguchi, A.; Peek, C.B.; Hong, H.; Huang, W.; Omura, C.; et al. Pancreatic β-cell Enhancers Regulate Rhythmic Transcription of Genes Controlling Insulin Secretion. *Science* **2015**, *350*, aac4250. [CrossRef]
21. Saad, A.; Man, C.D.; Nandy, D.K.; Levine, J.A.; Bharucha, A.E.; Rizza, R.A.; Basu, R.; Carter, R.E.; Cobelli, C.; Kudva, Y.C.; et al. Diurnal Pattern to Insulin Secretion and Insulin Action in Healthy Individuals. *Diabetes* **2012**, *61*, 2691–2700. [CrossRef]
22. van Cauter, E.; Blackman, J.D.; Roland, D.; Spire, J.-P.; Refetoff, S.; Polonsky, K.S. Modulation of glucose regulation and insulin secretion by circadian rhythmicity and sleep. *J. Clin. Investig.* **1991**, *88*, 934–942. [CrossRef]
23. Picinato, M.C.; Haber, E.P.; Carpinelli, A.R.; Cipolla-Neto, J. Daily rhythm of glucose-induced insulin secretion by isolated islets from intact and pinealectomized rat. *J. Pineal Res.* **2002**, *33*, 172–177. [CrossRef]
24. Sheets, A.R.; Fülöp, P.; Derdák, Z.; Kassai, A.; Sabo, E.; Mark, N.M.; Paragh, G.; Wands, J.R.; Baffy, G. Uncoupling protein-2 modulates the lipid metabolic response to fasting in mice. *Am. J. Physiol.-Gastrointest. Liver Physiol.* **2008**, *294*, 1017–1024. [CrossRef]
25. Affourtit, C.; Brand, M.D. On the role of uncoupling protein-2 in pancreatic beta cells. *Biochim. Biophys. Acta-Bioenerg.* **2008**, *1777*, 973–979. [CrossRef]
26. Boivin, D.B.; Boudreau, P. Impacts of shift work on sleep and circadian rhythms. *Pathol. Biol.* **2014**, *62*, 292–301. [CrossRef]
27. Karlsson, B.; Knutsson, A.; Lindahl, B. Is there an association between shift work and having a metabolic syndrome? Results from a population based study of 27 485 people. *Occup. Environ. Med.* **2001**, *58*, 747–752. [CrossRef]
28. Garaulet, M.; Gómes-Abellán, P.; Alburquerque-Béjar, J.J.; Lee, Y.-C.; Ordovás, J.M.; Scheer, F.A. Timing of food intake predicts weight loss effectiveness Prof. *Int. J. Obes.* **2013**, *37*, 604–611. [CrossRef]
29. Hatori, M.; Vollmers, C.; Zarrinpar, A.; DiTacchio, L.; Bushong, E.A.; Gill, S.; Leblanc, M.; Chaix, A.; Joens, M.; Fitzpatrick, J.A.; et al. Time-restricted feeding without reducing caloric intake prevents metabolic diseases in mice fed a high-fat diet. *Cell Metab.* **2012**, *15*, 848–860. [CrossRef]
30. Chaix, A.; Zarrinpar, A.; Miu, P.; Panda, S. Time-restricted feeding is a preventative and therapeutic intervention against diverse nutritional challenges. *Cell Metab.* **2014**, *20*, 991–1005. [CrossRef]
31. Tuomi, T.; Nagorny, C.L.F.; Singh, P.; Bennet, H.; Yu, Q.; Alenkvist, I.; Isomaa, B.; Östman, B.; Söderström, J.; Pesonen, A.-K.; et al. Increased Melatonin Signaling Is a Risk Factor for Type 2 Diabetes. *Cell Metab.* **2016**, *23*, 1067–1077. [CrossRef]
32. Marrone, G.; Guerriero, C.; Palazzetti, D.; Lido, P.; Marolla, A.; Di Daniele, F.; Noce, A. Vegan diet health benefits in metabolic syndrome. *Nutrients* **2021**, *13*, 817. [CrossRef]
33. Shapira, N. The metabolic concept of meal sequence vs. Satiety: Glycemic and oxidative responses with reference to inflammation risk, protective principles and mediterranean diet. *Nutrients* **2019**, *11*, 2373. [CrossRef]
34. Kahleova, H.; Hlozkova, A.; Fleeman, R.; Fletcher, K.; Holubkov, R.; Barnard, N.D. Fat quantity and quality, as part of a low-fat, vegan diet, are associated with changes in body composition, insulin resistance, and insulin secretion. A 16-week randomized controlled trial. *Nutrients* **2019**, *11*, 615. [CrossRef]
35. Mirabelli, M.; Chiefari, E.; Arcidiacono, B.; Corigliano, D.M.; Brunetti, F.S.; Maggisano, V.; Russo, D.; Foti, D.P.; Brunetti, A. Mediterranean Diet Nutrients to Turn the Tige against Insulin Resistance and Related Diseases. *Nutrients* **2020**, *12*, 1066. [CrossRef]
36. ROOT, H.F. Insulin resistance. *Pa. Med. J.* **1954**, *57*, 1098–1099.
37. Waldmann, A.; Ströhle, A.; Koschizke, J.W.; Leitzmann, C.; Hahn, A. Overall glycemic index and glycemic load of vegan diets in relation to plasma lipoproteins and triacylglycerols. *Ann. Nutr. Metab.* **2007**, *51*, 335–344. [CrossRef]
38. Rodríguez-Rejón, A.I.; Castro-Quezada, I.; Ruano-Rodríguez, C.; Ruiz-López, M.D.; Sánchez-Villegas, A.; Toledo, E.; Artacho, R.; Estruch, R.; Salas-Salvadó, J.; Covas, M.I.; et al. Effect of a Mediterranean Diet Intervention on Dietary Glycemic Load and Dietary Glycemic Index: The PREDIMED Study. *J. Nutr. Metab.* **2014**, *2014*, 985373. [CrossRef]
39. Chiu, T.H.T.; Pan, W.H.; Lin, M.N.; Lin, C.L. Vegetarian diet, change in dietary patterns, and diabetes risk: A prospective study. *Nutr. Diabetes* **2018**, *8*, 12. [CrossRef]
40. Kahleova, H.; Matoulek, M.; Malinska, H.; Oliyarnik, O.; Kazdova, L.; Neskudla, T.; Skoch, A.; Hajek, M.; Hill, M.; Kahle, M.; et al. Vegetarian diet improves insulin resistance and oxidative stress markers more than conventional diet in subjects with Type2 diabetes. *Diabet. Med.* **2011**, *28*, 549–559. [CrossRef]
41. Otten, J.; Ryberg, M.; Mellberg, C.; Andersson, T.; Chorell, E.; Lindahl, B.; Larsson, C.; Holst, J.J.; Olsson, T. Postprandial levels of GLP-1, GIP and glucagon after 2 years of weight loss with a Paleolithic diet: A randomised controlled trial in healthy obese women. *Eur. J. Endocrinol.* **2019**, *180*, 417–427. [CrossRef]
42. Schwingshackl, L.; Chaimani, A.; Hoffmann, G.; Schwedhelm, C.; Boeing, H. A network meta-analysis on the comparative efficacy of different dietary approaches on glycaemic control in patients with type 2 diabetes mellitus. *Eur. J. Epidemiol.* **2018**, *33*, 157–170. [CrossRef]
43. Manheimer, E.W.; van Zuuren, E.J.; Fedorowicz, Z.; Pijl, H. Paleolithic nutrition for metabolic syndrome: Systematic review and meta-analysis. *Am. J. Clin. Nutr.* **2015**, *102*, 922–932. [CrossRef]
44. Genoni, A.; Christophersen, C.T.; Lo, J.; Coghlan, M.; Boyce, M.C.; Bird, A.R.; Lyons-Wall, P.; Devine, A. Long-term Paleolithic diet is associated with lower resistant starch intake, different gut microbiota composition and increased serum TMAO concentrations. *Eur. J. Nutr.* **2020**, *59*, 1845–1858. [CrossRef]

45. Napoleão, A.; Fernandes, L.; Miranda, C.; Marum, A.P. Effects of calorie restriction on health span and insulin resistance: Classic calorie restriction diet vs. Ketosis-inducing diet. *Nutrients* **2021**, *13*, 1302. [CrossRef]
46. Rosenbaum, M.; Hall, K.D.; Guo, J.; Ravussin, E.; Mayer, L.S.; Reitman, M.L.; Smith, S.R.; Walsh, B.T.; Leibel, R.L. Glucose and Lipid Homeostasis and Inflammation in Humans Following an Isocaloric Ketogenic Diet. *Obesity* **2019**, *27*, 971–981. [CrossRef]
47. Grandl, G.; Straub, L.; Rudigier, C.; Arnold, M.; Wueest, S.; Konrad, D.; Wolfrum, C. Short-term feeding of a ketogenic diet induces more severe hepatic insulin resistance than an obesogenic high-fat diet. *J. Physiol.* **2018**, *596*, 4597–4609. [CrossRef]
48. Kothari, V.; Luo, Y.; Tornabene, T.; O'Neill, A.M.; Greene, M.W.; Geetha, T.; Babu, J.R. High fat diet induces brain insulin resistance and cognitive impairment in mice. *Biochim. Biophys. Acta-Mol. Basis Dis.* **2017**, *1863*, 499–508. [CrossRef]
49. Koh, J.-H.; Johnson, M.L.; Dasari, S.; Lebrasseur, N.K.; Vuckovic, I.; Henderson, G.C.; Cooper, S.A.; Manjunatha, S.; Ruegsegger, G.N.; Shulman, G.I.; et al. TFAM enhances fat oxidation and attenuates high-fat diet-induced insulin resistance in skeletal muscle. *Diabetes* **2019**, *68*, 1552–1564. [CrossRef]
50. Foley, P.J. Effect of low carbohydrate diets on insulin resistance and the metabolic syndrome. *Curr. Opin. Endocrinol. Diabetes Obes.* **2021**, *28*, 463–468. [CrossRef]
51. Feinman, R.D.; Pogozelski, W.K.; Astrup, A.; Bernstein, R.K.; Fine, E.J.; Westman, E.C.; Accurso, A.; Frassetto, L.; Gower, B.A.; McFarlane, S.I.; et al. Dietary carbohydrate restriction as the first approach in diabetes management: Critical review and evidence base. *Nutrition* **2015**, *31*, 1–13. [CrossRef]
52. Nicholls, J. Perspective: The Glycemic Index Falls Short as a Carbohydrate Food Quality Indicator to Improve Diet Quality. *Front. Nutr.* **2022**, *9*, 784. [CrossRef]
53. Jackson, K.H.; West, S.G.; Heuvel, J.P.V.; Jonnalagadda, S.S.; Ross, A.B.; Hill, A.M.; A Grieger, J.; Lemieux, S.K.; Kris-Etherton, P. Effects of whole and refined grains in a weight-loss diet on markers of metabolic syndrome in individuals with increased waist circumference: A randomized controlled-feeding trial. *Am. J. Clin. Nutr.* **2014**, *100*, 577–586. [CrossRef]
54. Ludwig, D.S.; Ebbeling, C.B. The carbohydrate-insulin model of obesity: Beyond 'calories in, calories out. *JAMA Intern. Med.* **2018**, *178*, 1098–1103. [CrossRef]
55. Pereira, M.A.; Jacobs, D.R., Jr.; Pins, J.J.; Raatz, S.K.; Gross, M.D.; Slavin, J.L.; Seaquist, E.R. Effect of whole grains on insulin sensitivity in overweight hyperinsulinemic adults. *Am. J. Clin. Nutr.* **2002**, *75*, 848–855. [CrossRef]
56. Malin, S.K.; Kullman, E.L.; Scelsi, A.R.; Haus, J.M.; Filion, J.; Pagadala, M.R.; Godin, J.-P.; Kochhar, S.; Ross, A.B.; Kirwan, J.P. A whole-grain diet reduces peripheral insulin resistance and improves glucose kinetics in obese adults: A randomized-controlled trial. *Metabolism* **2018**, *82*, 111–117. [CrossRef]
57. Herrmann, T.S.; Bean, M.L.; Black, T.M.; Wang, P.; Coleman, R.A. High glycemic index carbohydrate diet alters the diurnal rhythm of leptin but not insulin concentrations. *Exp. Biol. Med.* **2001**, *226*, 1037–1044. [CrossRef]
58. Joaquim, L.; Faria, A.; Loureiro, H.; Matafome, P. Benefits, mechanisms, and risks of intermittent fasting in metabolic syndrome and type 2 diabetes. *J. Physiol. Biochem.* **2022**, *78*, 295–305. [CrossRef]
59. Antoni, R.; Johnston, K.L.; Collins, A.L.; Robertson, M.D. Efects of intermittent fasting on glucose and lipid metabolism. *Proc. Nutr. Soc.* **2017**, *76*, 361–368. [CrossRef]
60. Réda, A.; Wassil, M.; Mériem, M.; Alexia, P.; Abdelmalik, H.; Sabine, B.; Nassir, M. Food timing, circadian rhythm and chrononutrition: A systematic review of time-restricted eating's efects on human health. *Nutrients* **2020**, *12*, 3770. [CrossRef]
61. Ye, Y.; Xu, H.; Xie, Z.; Wang, L.; Sun, Y.; Yang, H.; Hu, D.; Mao, Y. Time-restricted feeding reduces the detrimental efects of a high-fat diet, possibly by modulating the circadian rhythm of hepatic lipid metabolism and gut microbiota. *Front. Nutr.* **2020**, *7*, 596285. [CrossRef]

diabetology

MDPI

Review

Gut Metabolism of Sugars: Formation of Glycotoxins and Their Intestinal Absorption

Tamaeh Monteiro-Alfredo [1,2] and Paulo Matafome [1,2,3,4,5,*]

[1] Coimbra Institute for Clinical and Biomedical Research (iCBR) and Institute of Physiology, Faculty of Medicine, University of Coimbra, 3000-354 Coimbra, Portugal
[2] Center for Innovative Biomedicine and Biotechnology (CIBB), University of Coimbra, 3004-531 Coimbra, Portugal
[3] Clinical Academic Center of Coimbra (CACC), 3000-548 Coimbra, Portugal
[4] Department of Complementary Sciences, Instituto Politécnico de Coimbra, Coimbra Health School (ESTeSC), 3046-854 Coimbra, Portugal
[5] Faculty of Medicine, Pole III of University of Coimbra, Subunit 1, 1st Floor, Azinhaga de Santa Comba, Celas, 3000-354 Coimbra, Portugal
* Correspondence: paulo.matafome@uc.pt; Tel.: +351-239480014

Abstract: Glycotoxins include the group of advanced glycation end-products (AGEs) and their precursors, most of them highly reactive intermediary compounds of sugar metabolism. Glycotoxins and products of the Maillard reaction are present in high concentrations in foods rich in sugars and processed at high temperatures and are often associated with the flavour of the food. Proteins undergoing this type of molecular modification are targets for gut peptidases and may be absorbed into circulation. AGEs are associated with the toxic effects of glucose in diabetic patients, and some studies have shown that they also contribute to metabolically unhealthy obesity and prediabetes development. Restriction of dietary glycotoxins was shown to improve insulin resistance in humans. However, the real contribution of dietary AGEs to such mechanisms is still not understood. This review summarizes the current knowledge about glycotoxin formation from dietary sugars, their digestion throughout the gastrointestinal system, and the mechanisms of their intestinal absorption.

Keywords: glycation; glycotoxins; dietary sugars; AGEs digestion; intestinal absorption; gut microbiota

Citation: Monteiro-Alfredo, T.; Matafome, P. Gut Metabolism of Sugars: Formation of Glycotoxins and Their Intestinal Absorption. *Diabetology* **2022**, 3, 596–605. https://doi.org/10.3390/diabetology3040045

Academic Editor: Peter Clifton

Received: 9 October 2022
Accepted: 7 November 2022
Published: 10 November 2022

1. Introduction

Free sugars are often very reactive and are non-enzymatically degraded under physiological conditions, leading to the formation of intermediary compounds that may react with other molecules and cause harmful effects. This pool of intermediary and advanced products is generally called glycotoxins. This is a heterogeneous group of compounds that includes advanced glycation end-products (AGEs) and their precursors, most of them highly reactive intermediary compounds. Methylglyoxal (MG) is a dicarbonyl and a major precursor that originates as a by-product of glucose and fructose metabolism (reviewed by [1]). It modifies arginine and lysine residues of biomolecules, namely, proteins and DNA, forming AGEs [1–4]. The AGEs Nδ-(5-hydro-5-methyl-4-imidazolon-2-yl)-ornithine (MG-H1) and argpyrimidine are formed after MG-induced arginine modification, whereas lysine modification leads to methylglyoxal lysine dimer (MOLD) and (carboxyethyl)lysine (CEL) formation [5–8]. Alternatively, NE-(carboxymethyl)-lysine (CML), one of the major AGEs, may be formed directly from the Maillard reaction between lysine residues and reducing sugars, fructose being more harmful than glucose [1]. Such reactions may occur intracellularly (cytoplasmic proteins and transcription factors) or with circulating (haemoglobin, albumin, or lipoproteins) extracellular matrix and food proteins [1–4,9]. The endogenous formation of MG-derived AGEs has been associated with diabetes-like vascular and metabolic complications. Their contribution to nephropathy and retinopathy has been consistently shown, not only due to direct effects on endothelial cells but also on podocytes and pericytes. In the development of the diabetic foot, glycotoxins have been shown to contribute both to vascular dysfunction and neuropathy, leading to hypersensitivity of nerve fibres and neuronal degeneration (reviewed by [1,8]). They have also been shown to cause insulin resistance, mainly in already obese models and beta-cell dysfunction. Although a few reports show that their decrease in diet may reduce insulin resistance in diabetic patients, rodent models of AGEs supplementation fail to show insulin resistance. Otherwise, if AGE supplementation is made to high-fat diet-fed rodent models, they potentiate the diet's effects and trigger insulin resistance (reviewed by [10]). Glycotoxins and AGEs are well-known contributors to a myriad of other metabolic disease-related disorders. Their contribution has been shown in cardiovascular and cerebrovascular diseases due to endothelial dysfunction in macrovessels, alterations in cardiac muscle contractility/relaxation, tendon stiffness, and even rheumatoid arthritis. Glycotoxins have also been linked with the molecular mechanisms of central nervous system disorders, namely, mitochondrial dysfunction and oxidative stress in Alzheimer's disease and glycation of alpha-synuclein in Parkinson's disease (reviewed by [1,8,11]).

Modification of intracellular proteins by dicarbonyls like MG changes the cellular redox state (oxidative and nitrosative stress), proteasomal activity, and gene expression modulators, while modification of extracellular and circulating proteins leads to increased stiffness of the matrix and alteration of biological properties of circulating factors, such as hormone loss of function and modification of albumin and haemoglobin [1]. MG may be detoxified into D-lactate through the glyoxalase system (GLO-1 and GLO-2), while AGEs and their intermediary Amadori products, such as fructoselysine, may be cleared by amadoriases. Of those, the fructosyl amine oxidase (FAOX) amadoriase, it is the most well studied and characterized for its catalytic activity, cleaving the adducts between sugars and amino acids. Other enzymes include amadoriase II and other amadoriases occurring in other organisms (reviewed by [1,12]). The GLO system is GSH-dependent and its downregulation is associated with higher endogenous AGE formation and the development of diabetic complications in humans and animal models [8].

Despite their quantitative contribution to the circulating pool is not completely understood, glycotoxins may also originate in the diet, namely, in foods rich in sugars and cooked at high temperatures. Using human serum albumin as a model, the dicarbonyls glyoxal and methylglyoxal have been shown to modify the lysyl and arginyl groups in 9 and 14 sites, respectively [13]. Although this depends on each specific protein and the sugars involved, sugar-rich foods and cooking also lead to the initiation of similar reactions involving food proteins. Even in healthy individuals, circulating AGE levels are correlated with their intake, contributing to the endogenous pool of AGEs and activation of inflammatory signals [14–16]. Intestinal absorption of glycotoxins and AGEs has been shown, as well as their deposition in tissues [17]. In foods, the initial steps of the Maillard reaction originate from such Amadori products as fructoselysine and lactuloselysine and AGEs, which are estimated to be consumed on a scale of daily 500–1200 mg in the diet. About 25–75 mg are estimated to be AGEs. Pasteurized milk and bakery products are the main dietary sources of Amadori products [18,19]. However, the digestion and absorption processes are very different among distinct AGEs, imposing extra difficulties in their study.

Although AGEs may be absorbed from the diet, mainly through the Maillard reaction, in sugar-rich foods, there are also other components that may prevent such reactions. The presence of antioxidants and scavenging molecules may hamper AGE formation, although this is still mostly unknown ground. Nevertheless, pectin oligosaccharides were recently shown to prevent food browning (Maillard reaction) and inhibit AGE formation. This is a complex group of non-digestible oligosaccharides originating from pectin, present in the plant cell wall. These compounds also reduced intestinal absorption in an in vitro system, suggesting their use as a dietary supplement to prevent food glycation [20]. Another way to promote the detoxification of AGEs is through the ingestion of vegetables, fruits, and natural foods rich in phenolic compounds, which have anti-glycating [21] and antioxidant activity [22,23].

2. Formation of Glycotoxins in the Gut and Their Digestion

Advanced glycation end-product (AGE) formation during carbohydrate digestion: Carbohydrates can be found in the most varied sources: they can be intrinsic to fruit and milk or they can be added to food (extrinsic sugars) to increase palatability and conservation [24]. In recent times, the new habits of the world population are associated with a greater consumption of sugars and consequently AGEs. In general, AGEs provide greater palatability and help to increase shelf life [25]. Although food is an important exogenous source, they may also be produced during digestion, becoming an endogenous source of AGEs [14] (Figure 1). The energy value offered by sugar is 4 kcal g^{-1}, and the recommended intake of carbohydrates is based on the minimum amount of sugar consumed by the brain, which is 130 g day^{-1} for both adults and children [26]. Despite this, the actual consumption is above the recommended daily average, according to the Centers for Disease Control and Prevention [27]. The increased consumption of sugars is directly related to the development of obesity, type 2 diabetes, and associated pathologies [23].

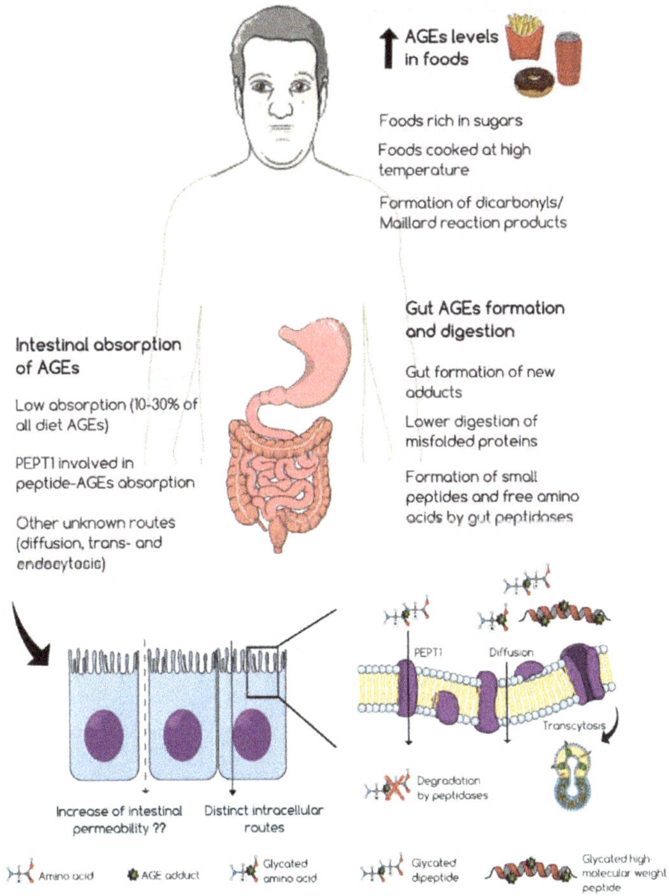

Figure 1. Overview of the events involved in glycotoxin consumption from sugar-rich foods, their digestion in the gastrointestinal tract, and their intestinal absorption. The lower part of the image shows the different mechanisms described to be involved in intestinal AGE absorption.

Carbohydrate digestion begins in the mouth with the entire physical and chemical process that occurs with the concomitant action of α-amylase and the subsequent effect of pancreatic amylase, located in the small intestine, which is responsible for the digestion of 60% of carbohydrates. Then, the monosaccharides are absorbed by enterocytes into the bloodstream through intestinal epithelial cell enzymes [28]. Finally, they are transferred to cells to participate in energy production, which can be aerobic or anaerobic [29], and are eventually oxidized [30]. As consequence of the exaggerated intake of sugars, the reactions that occur from glucose with the body's proteins give rise to dicarbonyls and AGEs, which gradually accumulate in the body. One of the sugar-driven modifications is the case of glycated haemoglobin (HbA1c), a biochemical marker of glycaemic control in diabetic patients, which reflects the mean glycaemia of the last 90 to 120 days [31].

In addition to the ingestion of exogenous AGEs, their formation can occur through chemical processes of food degradation. Diet-derived MG interacts with intestinal proteins and culminates in the formation of the derivative of arginine MG-H1, which is absorbed in the intestine by enterocytes [32]. In simulations of digestive conditions, the concentrations of these AGEs were reduced in the presence of pancreatic enzymes. Regarding MG, its stability is greater in the gastric juice, but its degradation occurs in the intestinal juice, which probably is related to an enzymatic action [33]. It is believed that the digestive characteristics of AGEs in general lead to their susceptibility to the metabolism of reversibly bound adducts during digestion, and may later promote some local or systemic effect if they are reabsorbed [34] (Figure 1).

For the digestion of AGEs, gastric and intestinal functions are critical and depend on the function of such enzymes as elastase, peptidases, trypsin, and chymotrypsin. Glycation of arginine and lysine residues may directly block the trypsin site (which occurs by the attraction of negative charges between the trypsin active centre (negatively charged) and the amino acid groups (positively charged), being responsible for the impairment of the protein digestive process. Additionally, this modification may also hinder the effect of other digestive proteases, such as β-lactoglobulin and β-casein [35]. On the other hand, in another study, it was confirmed that alterations in the conformation of lactoferrin, caused by glycation, can lead to greater exposure of cleavage sites, increasing susceptibility to proteolysis [36]. The anti-digestion profile of AGEs ends up functioning as a natural barrier against the absorption of AGEs that are bound to proteins, because they have a lower bioavailability than free fractions [37].

Other studies with mice revealed the formation of specific AGEs from dietary sugars, namely, the detection of AGEs derived from MG in the liver tissue after glucose intake, and the detection of glyoxal (GO) when ingesta were based on fructose [32]. A study carried out by Martínez-Saez [38], which aimed to define the products derived from the Maillard reaction from meals, determined that physiological concentrations of sugars (43 mM) already caused the formation of these products. Fructose at a concentration of 314 mM was able to promote the formation of fructosamine and other AGEs, and fructose at 43 mM with lysine was able to give rise to CML [38]. In another assay, where different products obtained from gastric and intestinal digestion were analysed, namely, CEL, CML, MG-H1, and hydroimidazolone 1 derived from GO (G-H1), the binding of these structures in the free form associated with proteins was observed, showing that the link between both survives after the gastrointestinal digestion process, in addition to having the ability of entering the human gastrointestinal tract and triggering a pro-inflammatory environment [39] (Figure 1).

Regarding conformational changes, dietary glycated proteins may naturally trigger changes that can play an important role in the digestion of these sets of glycated amino acids. Studies show that the non-cross-linked structures display a reduction in the digestibility of the glycated protein, as occurred with CML-casein. When submitted to a proteolysis procedure, its digestibility was considerably lower than the native casein [40]. This condition is probably associated with a reduction in molecular accessibility that allows the cleavage of the main chain of the protein. In this context, AGEs that have non-crosslinked structures, such as CMA, CML, and pyrraline, originate from the covalent alteration of residues of arginine and lysine, and because of this change, can cause trypsin blockage in the intestinal digestion process [9].

The role of gut microbiota and sugar/AGE metabolism: Several recent studies have brought evidence that relates the imbalance of the intestinal microbiota caused by the intake of sugars with insulin resistance, diabetes, obesity [41–43], and metabolic syndrome, by interrupting the immune-mediated protection necessary for body homeostasis [43]. Leptin-deficient ob/ob mice, for example, have a completely different microbial composition from normal mice, and the different taxa observed suggest the existence of a microbiota–host cross-talk that relates body composition to the metabolism of animals [42]. Although so far not many details are known about the metabolism of AGEs, there are reports regarding the probable action of the intestinal microbiota in this process, especially regarding Amadori products. This is based on a recent characterization of bacterial enzymes (fructoseamine-6-kinase) that allow the metabolism of these products by different bacteria, such as *Escherichia coli* [44].

In a study carried out by Mastrocola [45], it was reported that a diet enriched with MG-H1 can cause an increase in tissue AGEs, which culminated in an inflammatory imbalance and an alteration in the homeostasis of the intestinal microbiota. It has been proven that the faecal excretion of AGEs does not exceed 50%, and thus it is believed that AGEs are neither absorbed nor excreted and can be metabolized intraluminally by the intestinal microbiota itself. Bacteria such as *Anaerostipes*, *Candidatus Arthromitus*, *Bacteroidales_S24-7*, *Ruminococcus*, and *Prevotella*, among others, in general (not yet fully understood) are related to the maintenance of the immune system, regulation of the intestinal inflammatory process, insulin sensitization, have a direct relationship with metabolic diseases such as obesity and diabetes, and may undergo changes in their colonies due to the presence of AGEs in the gut [45]. Finally, in another study, this one carried out by Wang, in a trial where AGEs were also supplemented in the diet of animals, the authors also identified a negative change in *Bacteroidales_S24-7*, *Ruminococcaceae*, and related this condition with increased insulin resistance and a process of chronic inflammation [46].

3. Intestinal Absorption of Glycotoxins

Dietary AGE bioavailability: Whether dietary glycotoxins are absorbed at the intestinal level and contribute to the endogenous pool is still under debate, and several studies suggest that dicarbonyls and some AGEs may be scavenged and eliminated during digestion [47]. In studies carried out on humans, it was possible to detect mainly MG and GO after glucose intake [48]. However, in another human study carried out with a physiological intake of MG, it was not possible to detect MG or its metabolites in urine [33], suggesting that MG is possibly not absorbed into the bloodstream [32]. However, questions also remain about the methods to measure AGEs and their intermediaries in the circulation. Although several antibodies and kits are available for specific AGEs, they require further validation, because the epitope is an adduct and not an amino acid sequence. Even more complicated is the detection of intermediaries like carbonyls. For instance, MG detection is often made by high-performance liquid chromatography after derivatization. In fact, the most reliable method is mass spectrometry, as stated by Schalkwijk in his work (reviewed by [8]).

About 80% of all Amadori products are degraded by the intestinal flora and do not become AGEs. Moreover, recent evidence suggests that, of all AGEs in the diet, only about 10% are absorbed into the circulation and at least about 30% of these are excreted by urine, being this excretion percentage is higher for free AGEs than peptide-bound AGEs [16]. This was recently observed for the commonly found AGEs CEL, CML, and MG-H1 [49,50]. In animal models, CML accumulation in tissues was observed after consumption of an AGE-enriched diet. Higher concentrations were observed in the kidney, intestine, and lungs (81–320 μg CML g^{-1} dry matter), although it was also found in cardiac tissues, muscle, liver, and tendons [9]. Nevertheless, other studies did not find any correlation between dietary AGEs and free and peptide-bound AGEs in circulation [16]. The percentage of urinary recovery varies according to the type of AGE and the individual/model studied. For instance, faecal excretion of dietary CML was shown to be related to its dietary intake in adolescents, but its urinary excretion apparently has a progressive saturation [15]. Dietary pyrraline was described to be recovered in 50% in urine samples, while the free form of fluorescent AGE pentosine was found in up to 60% in urine after ingestion. For peptide-bound pentosane, the urinary recovery was much lower [51]. Free AGEs/glycated amino acids and protein-bound AGEs have distinct bioavailability and their renal excretion may vary according to several factors, such as kidney function, which is often compromised in diabetic patients. In healthy subjects, free AGEs are excreted much more, in part because protein-bound AGEs are reabsorbed in the proximal tubule, although it is also expected that their filtration rate could also be different [16]. However, such mechanisms may be completely different in patients with chronic kidney disease. In both healthy subjects and patients, these measures do not really inform about intestinal absorption, since AGEs may suffer conversion in the gut or after absorption or may simply be retained in tissue.

Mechanisms of dietary AGE absorption: Glycated peptides in general have much less affinity to membrane transporters than native amino acids [9]. Free and peptide-bound AGEs are likely to have distinct intestinal absorption mechanisms. AGEs bound to low-molecular-weight peptides like dipeptides were shown to be absorbed by the peptide transporter (PEPT1). These peptide-bound AGEs are later degraded by peptidases inside the enteric cells, appearing as free AGEs on the basolateral side [52] (Figure 1). This was observed, for instance, for pyrraline linked to alanine, but is less observed for other AGEs, suggesting that these mechanisms are AGE-specific [53]. AGEs bound to high-molecular-weight peptides, such as CML, argpyrimidine, or MG-H1, are most likely absorbed by simple diffusion, because they were shown not to inhibit the transport of endogenous ligands of the transporters, namely lysine transporters [54]. This type of AGE needs previous intestinal degradation before absorption, although hydrophobic AGEs like argpyrimidine were shown to pass the intestinal barrier more easily [52]. Transcytosis is also an alternative route of absorption for this type of AGE, although it is not expected to account for the major number of AGEs absorbed. A recent report on *C. elegans* showed that dietary CML may be effectively absorbed by endocytosis in the intestine wall [55]. Interestingly, free AGEs (single modified amino acids) were also shown to be poorly absorbed by peptide transporters and were suggested to be absorbed in low contents by simple diffusion [52]. It may be hypothesized that AGEs have different routes for absorption, considering not only their size but also their hydrophobicity and charge. It is also of note that lumen peptidase may have a role in preventing AGE absorption by cleaving peptides into single amino acids, which have been consistently shown to be poorly absorbed [37]. Furthermore, changes in protein conformation resulting, for instance, from cooking may alter these mechanisms, although further studies are necessary. One main concern about the absorption studies is that some of them are performed in cultured monolayer CACO-2 cells, which may not properly mimic in vivo conditions. Not only the transport system of these cells may be different but also the intracellular machinery responsible for AGE hydrolysis, which has major relevance for their absorption. Another major concern regarding the impact of dietary AGEs is that intestinal permeability has been shown to be increased in metabolic disorders and to be potentiated by poor dietary habits. It is possible that a significant number of dietary AGEs may be absorbed by intercellular transport due to a decrease in barrier integrity, while this is yet to be studied.

Inhibition of AGE intestinal absorption: As mentioned, foods rich in antioxidants and scavenging molecules may prevent intestinal absorption of Maillard reaction products and specific AGEs. However, specific products from the diet can directly inhibit AGE absorption. As also mentioned, pectin oligosaccharides were shown to reduce intestinal AGE formation and absorption at least in in vitro systems [20]. Other compounds, such as catechins and chlorogenic acid, were recently shown to inhibit AGE absorption in vitro [21,56]. Gut microbiota are a major player in degrading many of the diet's nutrients and components, and AGEs are no exception. Recently, it was shown that *Lactococcus lactis* bacteria can degrade dietary CML, mainly through β-galactosidase activity, significantly reducing intestinal absorption in healthy volunteers [57]. Nevertheless, the knowledge about this topic is still scarce and the discovery of new compounds able not only to prevent gut AGE formation but also their absorption may be a promising research area toward the prevention of harmful effects. In fact, several compounds have been shown in the last few years to scavenge glycotoxins in vitro and some were tested in vivo. Of those molecules, aminoguanidine, pyridoxamine, NAC, resveratrol, and sulforaphane stand out. However, few reports suggest their action in clearing dietary glycotoxins (reviewed by [1,8,58]). Some of them are known activators of NRF2, suggesting that could have beneficial effects on gut anti-glycation defences, although no studies have been reported in this topic. Thus, more research is needed in order to identify molecules able to directly scavenge dietary glycotoxins or to promote their clearance by the gut microbiota.

4. Conclusions and Future Perspectives

Glycotoxins are a heterogeneous group of compounds that were initially observed to contribute to the development of diabetic complications due to their increased endogenous formation from glucose. Later, data revealed their increased formation and accumulation in tissues, since earlier stages of the disease result from the dysregulated activity of detoxification systems and increased dietary consumption, namely, from high-glucose and high-fructose foods processed at high temperatures.

Despite the little information obtained so far, we have brought here what we already have about the deleterious effect of AGEs and the glycation of target molecules on the whole that involves the process of metabolizing AGEs in the GUT and the triggering of metabolic diseases, immunological and inflammation and nutritional homeostasis. Additionally, the microbial fraction also has incredible importance regarding the molecules absorbed, and the presence of certain strains is often mandatory for the development of physiological and pathological processes.

Its intestinal absorption seems to be AGE-dependent and is apparently more facilitated by AGEs linked to small peptides through peptide transporters. Other routes of absorption have also been suggested for free AGEs and AGEs linked to high-molecular-weight peptides, although their true role in the in vivo absorption of dietary AGEs is still to be proven. Nevertheless, the presence of dietary AGEs in circulation and urine is constant in several studies and the mechanisms of passage through the intestinal barrier should be addressed in the future. Additionally, the identification of molecules able to prevent their absorption may be of significance to reduce their biological impact.

Author Contributions: Conceptualization: T.M.-A. and P.M. Methodology: T.M.-A.; and P.M. Writing—original draft preparation: T.M.-A. and P.M. Writing—review and editing: P.M.; Supervision: P.M. All authors have read and agreed to the published version of the manuscript.

Funding: This work was supported by Foundation for Science and Technology (FCT), Portugal (PEst UID/NEU/04539/2013 and UID/NEU/04539/2019: CNC.IBILI; PEst UIDB/04539/2020 and UIDP/04539/2020: CIBB).

Institutional Review Board Statement: Not applicable.

Informed Consent Statement: Not applicable.

Data Availability Statement: The data presented in this study are available on request from the corresponding author.

Conflicts of Interest: The authors declare no conflict of interest.

Abbreviations

AGEs	advanced glycation end-products
CEL	(carboxyethyl)lysine
CMA	pg 8 só
CML	NE-(carboxymethyl)-lysine
G-H1	hydroimidazolone 1 derived from glyoxal

GLO	glyoxalase system
GO	glyoxal
MG	methylglyoxal
MG-H1	Nδ-(5-hydro-5-methyl-4-imidazolon-2-yl)-ornithine
MOLD	methylglyoxal lysine dimer
PEPT1	peptide transporter

References

1. Matafome, P.; Rodrigues, T.; Sena, C.; Seiça, R. Methylglyoxal in Metabolic Disorders: Facts, Myths, and Promises. *Med. Res. Rev.* **2017**, *37*, 368–403. [CrossRef] [PubMed]
2. Allaman, I.; Bélanger, M.; Magistretti, P.J. Methylglyoxal, the dark side of glycolysis. *Front. Neurosci.* **2015**, *9*, 23. [CrossRef] [PubMed]
3. Kalapos, M.P. Where does plasma methylglyoxal originate from? *Diabetes Res. Clin. Pract.* **2013**, *99*, 260–271. [CrossRef]
4. Poulsen, M.W.; Hedegaard, R.V.; Andersen, J.M.; de Courten, B.; Bügel, S.; Nielsen, J.; Skibsted, L.H.; Dragsted, L.O. Advanced glycation endproducts in food and their effects on health. *Food Chem. Toxicol.* **2013**, *60*, 10–37. [CrossRef] [PubMed]
5. Baynes, J.W.; Thorpe, S.R. Glycoxidation and lipoxidation in atherogenesis. *Free Radic. Biol. Med.* **2000**, *28*, 1708–1716. [CrossRef]
6. Kumagai, T.; Nangaku, M.; Kojima, I.; Nagai, R.; Ingelfinger, J.R.; Miyata, T.; Fujita, T.; Inagi, R. Glyoxalase I overexpression ameliorates renal ischemia-reperfusion injury in rats. *Am. J. Physiol. Renal Physiol.* **2009**, *296*, F912–F921. [CrossRef]
7. Roberts, M.J.; Wondrak, G.T.; Laurean, D.C.; Jacobson, M.K.; Jacobson, E.L. DNA damage by carbonyl stress in human skin cells. *Mutat. Res. Mol. Mech. Mutagen.* **2003**, *522*, 45–56. [CrossRef]
8. Schalkwijk, C.; Stehouwer, C.D.A. Methylglyoxal, a Highly Reactive Dicarbonyl Compound, in Diabetes, Its Vascular Complications, and Other Age-Related Diseases. *Physiol. Rev.* **2020**, *100*, 407–461. [CrossRef]
9. Liang, Z.; Chen, X.; Li, L.; Li, B.; Yang, Z. The fate of dietary advanced glycation end products in the body: From oral intake to excretion. *Crit. Rev. Food Sci. Nutr.* **2020**, *60*, 3475–3491. [CrossRef]
10. Matafome, P. Another Player in the Field: Involvement of Glycotoxins and Glycosative Stress in Insulin Secretion and Resistance. *Diabetology* **2020**, *1*, 24–36. [CrossRef]
11. Frolova, N.; Soboleva, A.; Nguyen, V.D.; Kim, A.; Ihling, C.; Eisenschmidt-Bönn, D.; Mamontova, T.; Herfurth, U.M.; Wessjohann, L.A.; Sinz, A.; et al. Probing glycation potential of dietary sugars in human blood by an integrated in vitro approach. *Food Chem.* **2021**, *347*, 128951. [CrossRef] [PubMed]
12. Almajwal, A.M.; Alam, I.; Abulmeaty, M.; Razak, S.; Pawelec, G.; Alam, W. Intake of dietary advanced glycation end products influences inflammatory markers, immune phenotypes, and antiradical capacity of healthy elderly in a little-studied population. *Food Sci. Nutr.* **2020**, *8*, 1046–1057. [CrossRef] [PubMed]
13. Delgado-Andrade, C.; Tessier, F.J.; Niquet-Leridon, C.; Seiquer, I.; Navarro, M.P. Study of the urinary and faecal excretion of N ε-carboxymethyllysine in young human volunteers. *Amino Acids* **2012**, *43*, 595–602. [CrossRef] [PubMed]
14. Nie, C.; Li, Y.; Qian, H.; Ying, H.; Wang, L. Advanced glycation end products in food and their effects on intestinal tract. *Crit. Rev. Food Sci. Nutr.* **2022**, *62*, 3103–3115. [CrossRef] [PubMed]
15. Delgado-Andrade, C.; Fogliano, V. Dietary Advanced Glycosylation End-Products (dAGEs) and Melanoidins Formed through the Maillard Reaction: Physiological Consequences of their Intake. *Annu. Rev. Food Sci. Technol.* **2018**, *9*, 271–291. [CrossRef] [PubMed]
16. Henle, T. AGEs in foods: Do they play a role in uremia? *Kidney Int.* **2003**, *63*, S145–S147. [CrossRef]
17. Henle, T. Protein-bound advanced glycation endproducts (AGEs) as bioactive amino acid derivatives in foods. *Amino Acids* **2005**, *29*, 313–322. [CrossRef] [PubMed]
18. Zhu, R.; Sun, X.; Zhang, Y.; Yang, T.; Wang, C.; Zhang, J.; Duan, Z.; Shang, F.; Fan, J.; Liu, Y.; et al. Effect of pectin oligosaccharides supplementation on infant formulas: The storage stability, formation and intestinal absorption of advanced glycation end products. *Food Chem.* **2022**, *373*, 131571. [CrossRef]
19. Bains, Y.; Gugliucci, A.; Caccavello, R. Advanced glycation endproducts form during ovalbumin digestion in the presence of fructose: Inhibition by chlorogenic acid. *Fitoterapia* **2017**, *120*, 1–5. [CrossRef]
20. Monteiro-Alfredo, T.; Oliveira, S.; Amaro, A.; Rosendo-Silva, D.; Antunes, K.; Pires, A.S.; Teixo, R.; Abrantes, A.M.; Botelho, M.F.; Castelo-Branco, M.; et al. Hypoglycaemic and Antioxidant Properties of *Acrocomia aculeata* (Jacq.) Lodd Ex Mart. Extract Are Associated with Better Vascular Function of Type 2 Diabetic Rats. *Nutrients* **2021**, *13*, 2856. [CrossRef]
21. Monteiro-Alfredo, T.; Caramelo, B.; Arbeláez, D.; Amaro, A.; Barra, C.; Silva, D.; Oliveira, S.; Seiça, R.; Matafome, P. Distinct Impact of Natural Sugars from Fruit Juices and Added Sugars on Caloric Intake, Body Weight, Glycaemia, Oxidative Stress and Glycation in Diabetic Rats. *Nutrients* **2021**, *13*, 2956. [CrossRef] [PubMed]
22. Slavin, J.; Carlson, J. Carbohydrates. *Adv. Nutr.* **2014**, *5*, 760–761. [CrossRef] [PubMed]
23. Uribarri, J.; Cai, W.; Woodward, M.; Tripp, E.; Goldberg, L.; Pyzik, R.; Yee, K.; Tansman, L.; Chen, X.; Mani, V.; et al. Elevated Serum Advanced Glycation Endproducts in Obese Indicate Risk for the Metabolic Syndrome: A Link Between Healthy and Unhealthy Obesity? *J. Clin. Endocrinol. Metab.* **2015**, *100*, 1957–1966. [CrossRef]
24. Ryan-Harshman, M.; Aldoori, W. New Dietary Reference Intakes for Macronutrients and Fibre. *Can Fam Physician* **2006**, *52*, 177–179.
25. CDC. Know Your Limit for Added Sugars. Available online: https://www.cdc.gov/nutrition/data-statistics/added-sugars.html (accessed on 21 September 2022).

26. Dashty, M. A quick look at biochemistry: Carbohydrate metabolism. *Clin. Biochem.* **2013**, *46*, 1339–1352. [CrossRef] [PubMed]
27. Erichsen, J.M.; Fadel, J.R.; Reagan, L.P. Peripheral versus central insulin and leptin resistance: Role in metabolic disorders, cognition, and neuropsychiatric diseases. *Neuropharmacology* **2022**, *203*, 108877. [CrossRef]
28. Tappy, L. Metabolism of sugars: A window to the regulation of glucose and lipid homeostasis by splanchnic organs. *Clin. Nutr.* **2021**, *40*, 1691–1698. [CrossRef] [PubMed]
29. Nagai, R.; Shirakawa, J.-I.; Fujiwara, Y.; Ohno, R.-I.; Moroishi, N.; Sakata, N.; Nagai, M. Detection of AGEs as markers for carbohydrate metabolism and protein denaturation. *J. Clin. Biochem. Nutr.* **2014**, *55*, 1–6. [CrossRef]
30. Hellwig, M.; Gensberger-Reigl, S.; Henle, T.; Pischetsrieder, M. Food-derived 1,2-dicarbonyl compounds and their role in diseases. Semin. *Cancer Biol.* **2018**, *49*, 1–8. [CrossRef]
31. Degen, J.; Vogel, M.; Richter, D.; Hellwig, M.; Henle, T. Metabolic Transit of Dietary Methylglyoxal. *J. Agric. Food Chem.* **2013**, *61*, 10253–10260. [CrossRef]
32. Papetti, A.; Mascherpa, D.; Gazzani, G. Free α-dicarbonyl compounds in coffee, barley coffee and soy sauce and effects of in vitro digestion. *Food Chem.* **2014**, *164*, 259–265. [CrossRef] [PubMed]
33. Zhao, D.; Li, L.; Le, T.T.; Larsen, L.B.; Su, G.; Liang, Y.; Li, B. Digestibility of Glyoxal-Glycated β-Casein and β-Lactoglobulin and Distribution of Peptide-Bound Advanced Glycation End Products in Gastrointestinal Digests. *J. Agric. Food Chem.* **2017**, *65*, 5778–5788. [CrossRef] [PubMed]
34. Moscovici, A.M.; Joubran, Y.; Briard-Bion, V.; Mackie, A.; Dupont, D.; Lesmes, U. The impact of the Maillard reaction on the in vitro proteolytic breakdown of bovine lactoferrin in adults and infants. *Food Funct.* **2014**, *5*, 1898–1908. [CrossRef] [PubMed]
35. Zhao, D.; Sheng, B.; Wu, Y.; Li, H.; Xu, D.; Nian, Y.; Mao, S.; Li, C.; Xu, X.; Zhou, G. Comparison of Free and Bound Advanced Glycation End Products in Food: A Review on the Possible Influence on Human Health. *J. Agric. Food Chem.* **2019**, *67*, 14007–14018. [CrossRef] [PubMed]
36. Martinez-Saez, N.; Fernandez-Gomez, B.; Cai, W.; Uribarri, J.; del Castillo, M.D. In vitro formation of Maillard reaction products during simulated digestion of meal-resembling systems. *Food Res. Int.* **2019**, *118*, 72–80. [CrossRef]
37. van der Lugt, T.; Venema, K.; van Leeuwen, S.; Vrolijk, M.F.; Opperhuizen, A.; Bast, A. Gastrointestinal digestion of dietary advanced glycation endproducts using anin vitromodel of the gastrointestinal tract (TIM-1). *Food Funct.* **2020**, *11*, 6297–6307. [CrossRef]
38. Hellwig, M.; Matthes, R.; Peto, A.; Löbner, J.; Henle, T. N-ε-fructosyllysine and N-ε-carboxymethyllysine, but not lysinoalanine, are available for absorption after simulated gastrointestinal digestion. *Amino Acids* **2014**, *46*, 289–299. [CrossRef]
39. Heianza, Y.; Sun, D.; Li, X.; DiDonato, J.A.; Bray, G.A.; Sacks, F.M.; Qi, L. Gut microbiota metabolites, amino acid metabolites and improvements in insulin sensitivity and glucose metabolism: The POUNDS Lost trial. *Gut* **2019**, *68*, 263–270. [CrossRef]
40. Kashani, A.; Brejnrod, A.D.; Jin, C.; Kern, T.; Madsen, A.N.; Holm, L.A.; Gerber, G.K.; Holm, J.-C.; Hansen, T.; Holst, B.; et al. Impaired glucose metabolism and altered gut microbiome despite calorie restriction of ob/ob mice. *Anim. Microbiome* **2019**, *1*, 11. [CrossRef]
41. Kawano, Y.; Edwards, M.; Huang, Y.; Bilate, A.M.; Araujo, L.P.; Tanoue, T.; Atarashi, K.; Ladinsky, M.S.; Reiner, S.L.; Wang, H.H.; et al. Microbiota imbalance induced by dietary sugar disrupts immune-mediated protection from metabolic syndrome. *Cell* **2022**, *185*, 3501–3519.e20. [CrossRef]
42. Morales, F.J.; Somoza, V.; Fogliano, V. Physiological relevance of dietary melanoidins. *Amino Acids* **2012**, *42*, 1097–1109. [CrossRef] [PubMed]
43. Mastrocola, R.; Collotta, D.; Gaudioso, G.; Le Berre, M.; Cento, A.; Ferreira, G.A.; Chiazza, F.; Verta, R.; Bertocchi, I.; Manig, F.; et al. Effects of Exogenous Dietary Advanced Glycation End Products on the Cross-Talk Mechanisms Linking Microbiota to Metabolic Inflammation. *Nutrients* **2020**, *12*, 2497. [CrossRef]
44. Wang, J.; Cai, W.; Yu, J.; Liu, H.; He, S.; Zhu, L.; Xu, J. Dietary Advanced Glycation End Products Shift the Gut Microbiota Composition and Induce Insulin Resistance in Mice. *Diabetes Metab. Syndr. Obes.* **2022**, *15*, 427–437. [CrossRef] [PubMed]
45. Amoroso, A.; Maga, G.; Daglia, M. Cytotoxicity of α-dicarbonyl compounds submitted to in vitro simulated digestion process. *Food Chem.* **2013**, *140*, 654–659. [CrossRef]
46. Maessen, D.E.; Hanssen, N.M.; Scheijen, J.L.; van der Kallen, C.J.; van Greevenbroek, M.M.; Stehouwer, C.D.; Schalkwijk, C.G. Post–Glucose Load Plasma α-Dicarbonyl Concentrations Are Increased in Individuals with Impaired Glucose Metabolism and Type 2 Diabetes: The CODAM Study. *Diabetes Care* **2015**, *38*, 913–920. [CrossRef] [PubMed]
47. Palaseweenun, P.; Hagen-Plantinga, E.A.; Schonewille, J.T.; Koop, G.; Butre, C.; Jonathan, M.; Wierenga, P.A.; Hendriks, W.H. Urinary excretion of advanced glycation end products in dogs and cats. *J. Anim. Physiol. Anim. Nutr.* **2021**, *105*, 149–156. [CrossRef]
48. Scheijen, J.L.; Hanssen, N.M.; Van Greevenbroek, M.M.; Van Der Kallen, C.J.; Feskens, E.J.; Stehouwer, C.D.; Schalkwijk, C.G. Dietary intake of advanced glycation endproducts is associated with higher levels of advanced glycation endproducts in plasma and urine: The CODAM study. *Clin. Nutr.* **2018**, *37*, 919–925. [CrossRef]
49. Forster, S.; Gariballa, S. Age as a determinant of nutritional status: A cross sectional study. *Nutr. J.* **2005**, *4*, 28. [CrossRef]
50. Hellwig, M.; Geissler, S.; Matthes, R.; Peto, A.; Silow, C.; Brandsch, M.; Henle, T. Transport of Free and Peptide-Bound Glycated Amino Acids: Synthesis, Transepithelial Flux at Caco-2 Cell Monolayers, and Interaction with Apical Membrane Transport Proteins. *ChemBioChem* **2011**, *12*, 1270–1279. [CrossRef]
51. Hellwig, M.; Geissler, S.; Peto, A.; Knütter, I.; Brandsch, M.; Henle, T. Transport of Free and Peptide-Bound Pyrraline at Intestinal and Renal Epithelial Cells. *J. Agric. Food Chem.* **2009**, *57*, 6474–6480. [CrossRef]

52. Grunwald, S.; Krause, R.; Bruch, M.; Henle, T.; Brandsch, M. Transepithelial flux of early and advanced glycation compounds across Caco-2 cell monolayers and their interaction with intestinal amino acid and peptide transport systems. *Br. J. Nutr.* **2006**, *95*, 1221–1228. [CrossRef] [PubMed]
53. Dubois, C.; Litke, R.; Rianha, S.; Paul-Constant, C.; Guidice, J.-M.L.; Taront, S.; Tessier, F.J.; Boulanger, E.; Fradin, C. Exposure of Caenorhabditis elegans to Dietary Nε-Carboxymethyllysine Emphasizes Endocytosis as a New Route for Intestinal Absorption of Advanced Glycation End Products. *Nutrients* **2021**, *13*, 4398. [CrossRef] [PubMed]
54. Wu, Q.; Chen, Y.; Ouyang, Y.; He, Y.; Xiao, J.; Zhang, L.; Feng, N. Effect of catechin on dietary AGEs absorption and cytotoxicity in Caco-2 cells. *Food Chem.* **2021**, *355*, 129574. [CrossRef] [PubMed]
55. Park, H.-Y.; Lee, H.-B.; Lee, S.-Y.; Oh, M.-J.; Ha, S.K.; Do, E.; Lee, H.H.L.; Hur, J.; Lee, K.-W.; Nam, M.-H.; et al. Lactococcus lactis KF140 Reduces Dietary Absorption of Nε—(Carboxymethyl)lysine in Rats and Humans via β-Galactosidase Activity. *Front. Nutr.* **2022**, *9*, 916262. [CrossRef] [PubMed]
56. Rigoldi, F.; Spero, L.; Vedove, A.D.; Redaelli, A.; Parisini, E.; Gautieri, A. Molecular dynamics simulations provide insights into the substrate specificity of FAOX family members. *Mol. BioSyst.* **2016**, *12*, 2622–2633. [CrossRef]
57. Chegão, A.; Guarda, M.; Alexandre, B.M.; Shvachiy, L.; Temido-Ferreira, M.; Marques-Morgado, I.; Gomes, B.F.; Matthiesen, R.; Lopes, L.V.; Florindo, P.R.; et al. Glycation modulates glutamatergic signaling and exacerbates Parkinson's disease-like phenotypes. *NPJ Park. Dis.* **2022**, *8*, 51. [CrossRef]
58. He, C.; Sabol, J.; Mitsuhashi, T.; Vlassara, H. Dietary glycotoxins: Inhibition of reactive products by aminoguanidine facilitates renal clearance and reduces tissue sequestration. *Diabetes* **1999**, *48*, 1308–1315. [CrossRef]

diabetology MDPI

Review

Impact of Dietary Sugars on Gut Microbiota and Metabolic Health

Karina Garcia [1,2,3,4,†], Gonçalo Ferreira [1,2,3,†], Flávio Reis [1,2,3] and Sofia Viana [1,2,3,4,*]

1 Institute of Pharmacology & Experimental Therapeutics & Coimbra Institute for Clinical and Biomedical Research (iCBR), Faculty of Medicine, University of Coimbra, 3000-548 Coimbra, Portugal
2 Center for Innovative Biomedicine and Biotechnology (CIBB), University of Coimbra, 3004-504 Coimbra, Portugal
3 Clinical Academic Center of Coimbra (CACC), 3004-504 Coimbra, Portugal
4 Pharmacy, Coimbra Health School, Polytechnic Institute of Coimbra, Rua 5 de Outubro-SM Bispo, Apartado 7006, 3046-854 Coimbra, Portugal
* Correspondence: sofia.viana@uc.pt or sofia_viana@estesc.ipc.pt
† These authors contributed equally to this work.

Abstract: Excessive sugar consumption is a risk factor for the development of several disorders, including metabolic, cardiovascular, neurological conditions and even some cancers, and has been linked to increased morbidity and mortality. The popularization of the typical Western diet, featured by an excessive intake of saturated fats and added sugars and a low consumption of unprocessed fruits, vegetables and fiber, may directly affect the composition and functionality of the gut microbiota, staggering the balance of the intestinal microbiome that ultimately culminates into gut dysbiosis. Although added sugars in the form of nutritive and non-nutritive sweeteners are generally considered as safe, a growing body of evidence correlate their consumption with adverse effects on gut microbial ecosystem; namely an abnormal synthesis of short-chain fatty acids, altered intestinal barrier integrity and chronic inflammation that often fuel a panoply of metabolic conditions. Accordingly, this work revisited the available preclinical evidence concerning the impact of different types of dietary sugars—nutritive and non-nutritive sweeteners—on gut microbiota and metabolic health. Future research should consider gender and species vulnerability when the impact of such substances on GM community and metabolic health is scrutinized in order to guide their adequate use at doses relevant to human use.

Keywords: sugars; nutritive sweeteners; non-nutritive sweeteners; gut microbiota; metabolic health

Citation: Garcia, K.; Ferreira, G.; Reis, F.; Viana, S. Impact of Dietary Sugars on Gut Microbiota and Metabolic Health. *Diabetology* **2022**, 3, 549–560. https://doi.org/10.3390/diabetology3040042

Academic Editor: Medha Priyadarshini

Received: 17 September 2022
Accepted: 20 October 2022
Published: 28 October 2022

1. Introduction

Sugar consumption is increasing in a global scale with a negative impact on human health [1]. Sugars can be categorized as: (i) natural dietary sugars (e.g., glucose, fructose, sucrose), typically added as extrinsic sugars to foods and beverages during processing to sweeten and increase the flavor, being classified as nutritive sweeteners [2,3]; (ii) sugar alcohols (e.g., xylitol, sorbitol), also nutritive sweetener often used as alternatives to natural dietary sugars due to their low-caloric content [4]; and (iii) non-nutritive sweeteners (e.g., sucralose, saccharin) that, due to their noncaloric value, have gained popularity and are widely used in the scope of sugar reduction strategies [5,6].

The high consumption of dietary sugars is closely related with westernized diets, comprising highly processed foods and sugar-sweetened beverages that are strongly associated with an increased risk of poor health conditions [7–9]. For instance, sweetened foods display a key role for the development of dental caries, hyperactivity, obesity, diabetes, cardiovascular disease, hypertension, fatty liver disease, dyslipidemias and even some cancers [10–13]. Notably, a large number of abovementioned diseases display a gut dysbiotic scenario as well [14–17]. The overload of dietary sugar intake drives major changes in microbiota composition and function, namely a decreased bacterial diversity and altered metabolism that closely modulate epithelial integrity and gut inflammation [18–21]. Interestingly, gut dysbiotic scenarios driven by excessive sugar intake are strongly implicated in the development of dysmetabolic conditions, for instance metabolic syndrome, insulin resistance, dyslipidemia and type 2 diabetes and associated microvascular complications (e.g., nephropathy, retinopathy) [22–26]. Accordingly, this work aims to shed light to the impact of dietary sugars in GM composition and function and the ensuing effects in the metabolic health of the host.

2. Dietary Sugars—An Overview

Dietary sugars include distinct sources of sugars, which can be naturally occurring or added. The distinction between different types of sugars (i.e., total, free and naturally occurring) is crucial to best appreciate the association between sugar intake and health [27]. The World Health Organization (WHO) defines "free sugars" as all monosaccharides and disaccharides added to foods/beverages by the manufacturer, cook or consumption and sugars naturally present in honey, syrups, and fruit juices, including those concentrated [28,29]. The term "total sugars" refers to the combination of naturally occurring sugars and free sugars [29,30].

A healthy, well-balanced diet contains naturally occurring sugars present in fruits, vegetables, dairy products and many grains [31]. They can be in the form of simple molecules, monosaccharides (e.g., glucose, fructose, galactose) or disaccharides (e.g., sucrose, maltose, lactose), or more complex ones (e.g., polymers or polysaccharides) [32]. However, when these types of sugars are added as ingredients in processed foods to impart a sweet taste, they often correlate with excessive sugar intakes being associated with chronic disease conditions [33]. For example, fructose in the form of added sugar is particularly implicated in metabolic syndrome, hypertension, insulin resistance, lipogenesis, diabetes and associated retinopathy, kidney disease and inflammation [22–24]. Sucrose, glucose and fructose, when used in high amounts, have also a negative influence on oral hygiene and increase the risk of dental caries in children [34]. Therefore, WHO recommends in both adults and children a reduction in free sugars intake to less than 5–10% of total energy intake [29]. Furthermore, added sugars also comprise sweeteners-chemical compounds with an intrinsic sweet taste that determines their usage as sweetening agents [35,36]. Briefly, they can be classified due to their origin (natural or synthetic agents) or nutritional value (nutritive and non-nutritive) [37–39]. The structural formula of some nutritive and non-nutritive sweeteners is presented in Figure 1.

Nutritive sweeteners (NSs) enclose abovementioned carbohydrates (e.g., glucose sucrose, fructose) that provide approximately 4 kcal/g of energy and polyols (sugar alcohols), mostly hydrogenated carbohydrates that provide an average of 2 kcal/g of energy being often used as low-caloric sugar replacers [40]. Until now, several polyols have been approved to commercialization, such as xylitol (E967), maltitol (E953), sorbitol (E420), erythritol (E968), lactitol (E953) and mannitol (E421), to name just a few [41]. Such compounds elicit low glycemic and insulinemic responses due to the incomplete absorption from the small intestine into the blood stream. Moreover, they are also associated with lipogenesis inhibition [42]. However, since they are poorly absorbed in the colon, some laxative effects have been described and are not recommended for toddlers under 1 year of age [36,43].

Non-nutritive sweeteners (NNSs) or artificial sweeteners comprise substances with a great chemical diversity and a very intense sweet taste and offer little or no energy when ingested [32,44]. They are also known as high-intensity sweeteners since they are many times sweeter than sucrose. The most used NNSs are acesulfame potassium, aspartame, advantame, cyclamates, saccharin, sucralose, neohesperidin dihydrochalcone and neotame. Yet, some NNSs used in foods may also be isolated from natural sources, steviol glycosides, glycyrrhizin and thaumatin being some examples [40]. Notably, saccharin can have 300 times the potency of sucrose in terms of sweetening and has the acceptable daily intake (ADI) of 5 mg/kg of body weight. Aspartame and neotame display ADI values of

40 mg/kg and 18 mg/kg of body weight, respectively. However, due to their phenylalanine content, they are not advised for people with phenylketonuria [35,45]. Steviol glycosides are molecules extracted from the leaves of *Stevia rebaudiana* plant with an ADI limit of 4 mg/kg of body weight [46].

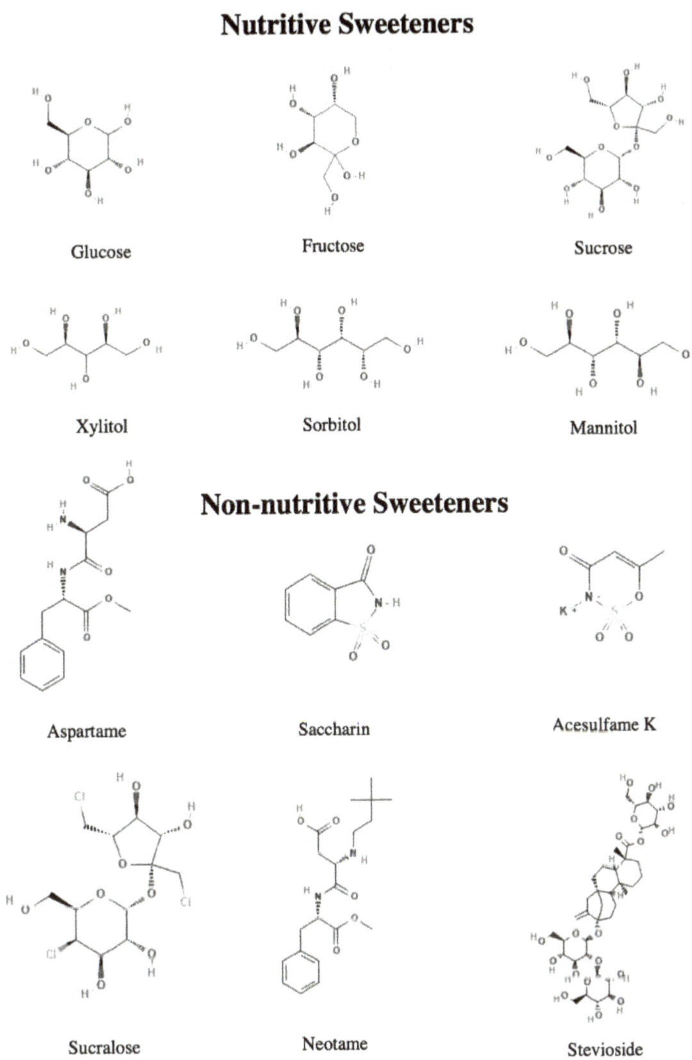

Figure 1. Nutritive and non-nutritive sweeteners chemical structures (Taken from: https://pubchem.ncbi.nlm.nih.gov/, accessed on 23 August 2022).

Even though NSs and NNSs are approved food additives that attempt to lower the overall daily caloric intake towards weight loss, concerns have emerged given their ability to modify the GM in such a way that there is the potential for an enhanced risk of glucose intolerance, insulin resistance, diabetes and increased weight [6,47,48].

3. Insights of Gut Microbiota Composition and Function

The term "microbiome", firstly utilized by Joshua Lederberg, has been gaining increasing importance, especially since 2001 [49]. Microbiome refers to a group of microorganisms living in a symbiotic way in our body. In a normal condition, the majority of GM is constituted by four main families: *Firmicutes* (64%), *Bacteroidetes* (23%), *Proteobacteria* (8%) and *Actinobacteria* (3%). Several studies recognize the key role of these bacteria in the extraction process of nutrients and energy from food as well as in human metabolism [50,51]. Accordingly, many researchers have depicted the deleterious impact of GM dysbiosis in the development of several host diseases [52]. For instance, the change in the GM composition in patients who have type 2 diabetes (T2D) is characterized by high levels of Streptococcus mutans, *Escherichia coli* and *Lactobacillus gasseri*, as well as by decreased levels of butyrate-producing bacteria such as *Clostridium Butyricum*, *Anaerostipes*, *Eubacterium halii*, *Roseburia* and *Faecalibacterium prauznitzii* [53]. Low *Firmicutes* abundance was also found in similar studies [54,55].

In addition, some metagenome-wide association studies support the idea that unbalanced intestinal environment can lead to the development of several diseases, affecting the integrity of the intestinal barrier, the production of short-chain fatty acids (SCFAs) and the metabolism of bile acids, among others [53]. SCFAs are metabolites produced by the microbial decomposition of nondigestible food and display chief roles for intestinal health [56]. Acetate (C2), propionate (C3) and butyrate (C4) are the most abundant SCFAs (60:20:20 ratio in the human gastrointestinal tract) [57]. Several studies have shown that an abnormal synthesis of SCFAs impact the integrity of intestinal barrier [58,59]. These microbial metabolites signal by distinct G protein-coupled receptors (GPRs), namely the GPR109a, GPR43 (FFAR2), GPR41 (FFAR3) and Olfactory receptor 78 [60]. Such receptors are expressed in several types of cells such as adipose, immune, hepatic or skeletal muscle cells [61,62]. Among all SCFAs, it has been reported that GPR41 receptor is activated by propionate, GPR43 receptor by propionate, acetate and butyrate and GPR109A receptor by butyrate [63–65]. In addition, several studies have shown that the activation of these receptors by SCFAs leads to the secretion of PYY (peptide tyrosine-tyrosine) into the colon with subsequent effects on central nervous system, namely appetite reduction [66]. Furthermore, the activation of GPR41 receptor stimulates the expression of leptin by adipocytes, resulting in the inhibition of neuropeptide Y (NPY) while the activation of GPR43 receptor leads to several positive effects, such as the suppression of glucagon from pancreatic α-cell or the release of GLP-1 (glucagon-like peptide-1) by endocrine L-cells who act in β-cell via stimulation of insulin biosynthesis and enhancement of glucose-stimulated insulin secretion [50,67].

Acetate is the most abundant SCFA in the gastrointestinal tract and several positive effects have been reported [68]. Den Besten and colleagues have shown that increased levels of acetate could improve insulin sensitivity, glucose homeostasis and reduce body weight [57,69]. However, other studies have shown contradictory evidence. For instance, a study from Perry and colleagues disclosed that high levels of acetate lead to the activation of parasympathetic nervous system, promoting an increased glucose stimulated insulin secretion and a higher production and secretion of ghrelin, resulting in weight gain [70,71].

Butyrate also displays important metabolic roles such as the activation of intestinal gluconeogenesis or macrophage M2 polarization towards anti-inflammatory effects through peroxisome proliferator-activated receptor gamma (PPARγ) up-regulation [72,73]. Furthermore, several studies have shown that the activation of this receptor also improves insulin sensitivity [74]. In addition, butyrate is also able to suppress NF-kB (nuclear factor kappa B) activation, an important transcription factor involved in the regulation of some genes encoding pro-inflammatory cytokines, growth factors, adhesion molecules, and immune receptors among others [75]. Several studies suggest that butyrate confers oxidative stress protection, regulates cell proliferation and cell differentiation, intestinal gluconeogenesis activation and maintains gut barrier permeability [76].

Remarkably, propionate supplementation was found to stimulate the release of the hormones PYY and GLP-1 in healthy adults resulting in a reduced appetite, hepatic fat, adipose tissue and a higher sensitivity to insulin [77]. Other studies also found the effects of propionate in Treg cells differentiation and production of interleukin (IL)-10 [78,79].

4. Impact of Dietary Sugars on Gut Microbiota and Metabolic Health

Several studies highlight the role of carbohydrates and sweeteners on satiety control, lipid metabolism, protein glycosylation, SCFAs production and the modulation of GM itself [80]. The ability of carbohydrates to modify the GM mostly relies on the non-digestible or digestible nature of these substrates [81]. Digestible carbohydrates such as sucrose or lactose are absorbed in the small intestine following degradation into monosaccharides (e.g., glucose, fructose) through a panoply of gastrointestinal enzymes [82]. Fructose, sugar alcohols and some non-nutritive sweeteners (e.g., sucralose) are passively, slowly or very poorly absorbed in the small intestine and overflow to the large intestine [2]. Such dynamics induce significant alterations in GM, including a reduced microbial diversity and altered relative abundance of certain bacterial phylum that correlates with metabolic health status, as highlighted in the following sections.

4.1. Nutritive Sweeteners

4.1.1. Glucose, Fructose, Sucrose

Consistent evidence from studies with animal models demonstrate that dietary patterns enclosing a high intake of glucose, fructose or sucrose lead to gut dysbiosis and metabolic imbalances, as summarized in Table 1. For example, in male C57BL/6J mice, the administration of a high-glucose diet (HGD) for 12 weeks elicited hyperglycemia, glucose intolerance, dyslipidemia and increased fat mass deposition [83]. In addition, the loss of gut microbial diversity, characterized by a lower proportion of Bacteroidetes and an increased proportion of Proteobacteria, has been observed [83]. Moreover, the HGD-fed animals displayed an increased gut permeability due to alterations in tight junction proteins as well as intestinal inflammation [83]. In the same study, similar results were noticed with the administration of a high-fructose diet (HfrD). Other authors also found that the administration of fructose at a low dose (2.6 g/kg/day), moderate dose (5.3 g/kg/day) and a high dose (10.5 g/kg/day) for 20 weeks leads to an increase in the serum pro-inflammatory cytokines (IL-6 and TNF-α: tumor necrosis factor-alpha) and a decrease in anti-inflammatory cytokine IL-10 in male Sprague Dawley rats. Notably, the higher fructose intake was associated to an increase abundancy of *Parasutterella* and *Blantia* and decreased *Intestinimonas* [84]. Furthermore, Sun and colleagues showed that male Wistar rats fed with a high-sucrose diet for 4 weeks significantly increased the serum triglycerides and cholesterol levels. Such changes were coincident with a scenario of gut dysbiosis, featured by an altered *Bacteroidetes/Firmicutes* ratio with an increase in Bacteroidetes and Verrucomicriobia and decreased Firmicutes [85].

4.1.2. Polyols

The relationship between polyols (also known as sugar alcohols) and GM composition and function has been also highlighted in distinct animal models. Xiang and colleagues reported no significant effects on pancreas, liver, brain and colon organ weights although it was observed increased levels of the GM metabolites butyrate and propionate in the intestinal mucosa and lumen of male C57BL/6 mice exposed to 2% (2.17 g/kg/day) and 5% (5.42 g/kg/day) of xylitol for 3 months. At the higher dose, xylitol elicited an increased abundance of *Bifidobacterium*, *Lactobacillus*, and *Erysipelotrichaceae* and decreased contents of *Blautia* and *Staphylococcus* [86]. Nevertheless, rodent species exhibit different susceptibilities as demonstrated by Zuo and colleagues who reported a decreased abundance of *Ruminococacaeae/Provotella* and increased *Bacteroides levels* in male Sprague Dawley rats but only when xylitol was administered at a higher-dose (xylitol 9.90 g/kg/day) [87].

Similarly, several studies demonstrated a disturbed GM upon sorbitol consumption. Accordingly, male Wistar rats exposed to 10% sorbitol (2.07 g/day) for 16 days showed an increase in *Lactobacillus abundance* and butyrate levels in the cecum and colon. Such changes paralleled lower levels of seric triglycerides, total cholesterol, HDL-cholesterol and LDL-cholesterol concentrations [88]. The consumption of 2% of lactitol also elicited a decrease in fecal pH and an increase in IgA hypersecretion in male Wistar rats without major differences in body weight curves [89]. Table 1 summarizes the alterations of GM composition and function upon polyols consumption.

Table 1. Effects of nutritive sweeteners on gut microbiota and metabolic health.

Intervention	Animal Model	Outcomes	Ref.
Administration of high-glucose and high-fructose diet (65.0% of calories in carbohydrate: 85% from glucose or fructose and 15% from sucrose) (12 weeks)	Male C57BL/6J mice	↑ Glucose intolerance and fasting blood glucose concentration ↑ Total and LDL cholesterol ↑ Serum endotoxin levels ↑ Proteobacteria, in particular Desulfovibrio vulgaris ↓ Bacteroidetes (Muribaculum intestinale) ↑ Akkermansia muciniphila ↓ ZO-1 and occludin expression in the colon ↑ Inflammatory cytokines, TNF-α and IL-1β, in the colon	[83]
Administration of fructose at low dose (Fru-L), (2.6 g/kg/day), moderate dose (Fru-M), (5.3 g/kg/day), high dose (Fru-H), (10.5 g/kg/day) (20 weeks)	Male Sprague Dawley rats	No significant differences in body weight and fasting blood glucose Fru-H ↑ Hepatic lipid accumulation and inflammatory cell infiltration in pancreas and colon ↑ Expression of lipid accumulation proteins (perilipin-1, ADRP, and Tip-47) in the colon ↑ Uric acid levels ↓ TJ proteins including ZO-1 and occludin ↑ Parasutterella and Blantia ↓ Intestinimonas Fru-L, Fru-M, Fru-H ↑ IL-6, TNF-α, and MIP-2 ↓ IL-10 ↓ isobutyric acid	[84]
High-sucrose diet (5.3 g sucrose/kg/day) (4 weeks)	Male Wistar rats	↑ Liver organ weight ↑ Serum triglycerides and cholesterol levels ↑ Hepatic lipids levels ↑ Bacteroidetes and Verrucomicriobia, Erysipelotrichaceae, Turicibacteraceae, Bacteroidaceae ↓ Firmicutes, Ruminococcaceae, Clostridiales, and Lactobacillacae	[85]
2% (2.17 g/kg/day), or 5% (5.42 g/kg/day) (*w*/*w*) xylitol (3 months)	Male C57BL/6 wild-type mice	No significant changes in brain, pancreas, colon and liver organ weights ↑ SCFA's, especially butyrate in the mucosa and propionate in the lumen 5% xylitol ↑ Bifidobacterium, Lactobacillus, and Erysipelotrichaceae ↓ Blautia and Staphylococcus	[86]
Approach	**Animal Model**	**Outcomes**	**Ref.**
Xylitol solution of 40 mg/kg and 200 mg/kg body weight/day (16 weeks)	Male C57B1/6J mice	Body composition, hepatic and serum lipid parameters, oral glucose tolerance were unaffected ↓ Bacteroidetes phylum and genus *Barnesiella*	[90]
1.0 g/100 kcal or 2.0 g/100 kcal of xylitol in the diet (8 weeks)	Diet-induced obese male Sprague Dawley rats	↓ Visceral fat mass, plasmatic insulin and lipid profile ↑ Fatty acid oxidation-related genes GM assessment was not evaluated	[91]
10% sorbitol (2.07 g/day) in water (16 days)	Male Wistar rats	↑ Colonic and cecal wall weights ↓ Serum lipid levels, triglycerides, total cholesterol, HDL-cholesterol and LDL-cholesterol ↑ Butyrate level in the cecum and colon ↑ *Lactobacillus* in feces, colon, cecum	[88]
2% (*w*/*w*) lactilol or 2% (*w*/*w*) polydextrose and lactilol (3 weeks)	Male Wistar rats	No differences in body weight No changes in the crypt:villus ratio ↑ IgA (lack of mucosal inflammation) ↑ Production of butyrate ↓ pH	[89]

4.2. Non-Nutritive Sweeteners

Likewise, a dysbiotic scenario has been reported upon the oral consumption of distinct non-nutritive sweeteners. Diet-induced obese male C57B1/6 mice presented impaired glucose tolerance and a reduction in *Lactobacillus reuteri* and an increase in fecal *Bacteroides* genus and Clostridiales order when 0.1 mg/mL of saccharin was administered for 10 weeks [92]. Similarly, the administration of 0.3 mg/mL saccharin for 6 months in male C57BL/6J mice triggered the hepatic overexpression of TNF-α and iNOS (Inducible nitric oxide synthase) along with an increase abundance of *Turicibacter Corynebacterium* and *Roseburia* and decreased contents of *Ruminococcus* and *Anaerostipes* [93]. In another study, an increase in Lactobacillus genus along with intraluminal lactic acid concentrations were observed in landrace X large white piglets fed with a diet supplemented with SUCRAM® 0.015% (*w*/*w*) saccaharin and neohesperidin dihydrochalcone for 2 weeks [94]. According to Abou-Donia and colleagues, the administration of 1.1, 3.3, 5.5 or 11 mg/kg/day of sucralose to Sprague Dawley rats for 12 weeks resulted in an increased body weight and a fewer number of *Bacteroides, Bifidobacterium, Clostridium* and *Lactobacilli* [95]. Yet, there are conflicting reports. For instance, the chronic administration of Acesulfame K solution (15 mg/kg/day) in male C57BL/6J mice did not elicit any significant change in GM composition. [96]. Nonetheless, Bian and colleagues have shown an increase in Bacteroides in male CD-1 mice fed with 37.5 mg/kg/day of Acesulfame-K along with an expressive body weight gain. Interestingly, these results were less pronounced in the female mice group, suggesting that gender differences must be taken into account [97]. In addition, aspartame and steviol glucosides are non-nutritive sweeteners that significantly disturb GM composition and function in obese and lactating rodents as well [98,99]. Table 2 outlines recent evidence focused on the impact of non-nutritive sweeteners on GM and metabolic health.

Table 2. Effects of non-nutritive sweeteners on gut microbiota and metabolic health.

Approach	Animal Model	Outcomes	Ref.
0.1 mg/mL saccharin in drinking water (10 weeks)	Diet-induced obese male C57Bl/6 Mice	Impaired glucose tolerance ↑ *Bacteroides* genus and Clostridiales order ↓ *Lactobacillus reuteri*	[92]
Oral dosing of Splenda (gavage) at 1.1, 3.3, 5.5 or 11 mg/kg/day sucralose (12 weeks)	Male Sprague Dawley rats	↑ Body weight ↓ *Bacteroides, bifidobacterium, lactobacilli* and *Clostridium* ↑ pH	[95]
Group 1: Administration of a high dose of sucralose (HS, 15 mg/kg body weight per day Group 2: Administration of Acesulfame K solution of 15 mg/kg body weight per day (8 weeks)	Male C57B1/6J mice	Group 1 ↑ Hepatic cholesterol concentration ↓ *Clostridium cluster XIVa* ↓ Butyrate concentration in cecal contents Group 2 GM was found unchanged	[96]
Oral dosing of Acesulfame K (gavage) at 37.5 mg/kg body weigh/day (4 weeks)	Male and female CD-1 mice	↑ Body weight (male mice only) ↑ *Bacteroides* (male mice group) ↓ *Lactobacillus* and *Clostridium* (female mice group)	[97]
High stevia diet (2.5% steviol glycosides) (Gestation and lactation period)	Female Wistar rats Male offspring (with standard diet)	↑ Fasting glucose levels of male offspring ↓ Bacteroides, Cyanobacteria ↑ Firmicutes, *Elusimicrobia, Lactobacillus*	[98]
Low-dose aspartame (5–7 mg/kg/day) in drinking water (8 weeks)	Diet-induced obese male Sprague Dawley rats	↓ Body fat percentage, insulin levels Fasting hyperglycemia and impaired insulin tolerance ↑ Enterobacteriaceae, *Clostridium leptum* ↑ Serum propionate	[99]
50 mg/kg/day of neohesperidin by gavage (4 groups: normal diet; normal diet + neo; High fat diet (HFD); HFD + neo) (12 weeks)	Male C57BL/6J mice	↓ Weight gain, dysfunctional glucose homeostasis, fatty liver, and systemic inflammation in HFD-fed mice ↑ Firmicutes ↓ Bacteroidetes (neo group)	[100]
0.75 mg/kg/day of neotame in drinking water (4 weeks)	Male CD-1 mice	No differences in body weight ↑ concentration of lipids and fatty acids in feces (linoleic acid, stearic acid, 1-monopalmitin and 1,3-dipalmitate) ↑ *Bacteroidetes phylum* ↓ Firmicutes, *Blautia, Dorea, Oscillospira* and *Ruminococcus* ↑ Microbial dysbiosis index	[101]

5. Conclusions

Reduction in the dietary intake of sugars has been strongly advised for some years now to cope with the prevention of non-communicable diseases such as diabetes, cardiovascular disease and/or obesity, among others. Accordingly, the use of alternative sweeteners, particularly those with a low-caloric content, has gained popularity. However, available preclinical evidence raises awareness on the dietary use of such substances in human health since they can also display putatively unfavorable effects on GM and metabolic health, as reviewed in this work. For instance, the decrease in SCFAs biosynthesis and intestinal barrier damage due to sweeteners-induced GM dysbiosis are well-described features of cardiovascular diseases, T2D and pancreatic damage, to name just a few [102–104].

Given the multifaceted roles of GM community in human health, future studies are warranted to provide adequate evidence regarding the impact of nutritive and non-nutritive sweeteners on metabolic status, with a major focus on gender and species vulnerability. Moreover, it would be of interest to further disclose key disease-altering properties of sweeteners and their candidate roles in nutrition therapy programs [105,106]. Such information will be paramount to guide their adequate use at doses relevant to human use.

Author Contributions: Conceptualization, S.V.; writing—original draft preparation, G.F. and K.G.; writing—review and editing, S.V., F.R. and K.G.; visualization, S.V. and F.R.; supervision, S.V. and F.R.; project administration, S.V. and F.R.; funding acquisition, S.V. and F.R. All authors have read and agreed to the published version of the manuscript.

Funding: This research was funded by National and European Funds, via Portuguese Science and Technology Foundation (FCT), European Regional Development Fund (FEDER), and Programa Operacional Factores de Competitividade (COMPETE): UIDP/04539/2020 (CIBB), PTDC/SAU-NUT/31712/2017, and POCI-01-0145-FEDER-031712.

Institutional Review Board Statement: Not applicable.

Informed Consent Statement: Not applicable.

Data Availability Statement: The data presented in this study are available on request from the corresponding author.

Conflicts of Interest: The authors declare no conflict of interest.

References

1. Stanhope, K.L. Sugar consumption, metabolic disease and obesity: The state of the controversy. *Crit. Rev. Clin. Lab. Sci.* **2016**, *53*, 52–67. [CrossRef] [PubMed]
2. Di Rienzi, S.C.; Britton, R.A. Adaptation of the Gut Microbiota to Modern Dietary Sugars and Sweeteners. *Adv. Nutr.* **2020**, *11*, 616–629. [CrossRef] [PubMed]
3. Heidari-Beni, M.; Kelishadi, R. The Role of Dietary Sugars and Sweeteners in Metabolic Disorders and Diabetes. In *Sweeteners: Pharmacology, Biotechnology, and Applications*; Mérillon, J.-M., Ramawat, K.G., Eds.; Springer International Publishing: Cham, Switzerland, 2018; pp. 225–243.
4. Hattori, K.; Akiyama, M.; Seki, N.; Yakabe, K.; Hase, K.; Kim, Y.G. Gut Microbiota Prevents Sugar Alcohol-Induced Diarrhea. *Nutrients* **2021**, *13*, 2029. [CrossRef]
5. Shankar, P.; Ahuja, S.; Sriram, K. Non-nutritive sweeteners: Review and update. *Nutrition* **2013**, *29*, 1293–1299. [CrossRef] [PubMed]
6. Liauchonak, I.; Qorri, B.; Dawoud, F.; Riat, Y.; Szewczuk, M.R. Non-Nutritive Sweeteners and Their Implications on the Development of Metabolic Syndrome. *Nutrients* **2019**, *11*, 644. [CrossRef] [PubMed]
7. Rodriguez-Ramirez, S.; Martinez-Tapia, B.; Gonzalez-Castell, D.; Cuevas-Nasu, L.; Shamah-Levy, T. Westernized and Diverse Dietary Patterns Are Associated with Overweight-Obesity and Abdominal Obesity in Mexican Adult Men. *Front. Nutr.* **2022**, *9*, 891609. [CrossRef] [PubMed]
8. Shi, Z. Gut Microbiota: An Important Link between Western Diet and Chronic Diseases. *Nutrients* **2019**, *11*, 2287. [CrossRef] [PubMed]
9. Garcia-Gutierrez, E.; Sayavedra, L. 3.07—Diet, Microbiota and the Gut-Brain Axis. In *Comprehensive Gut Microbiota*; Glibetic, M., Ed.; Elsevier: Oxford, UK, 2022; pp. 69–83.
10. Monteiro-Alfredo, T.; Caramelo, B.; Arbelaez, D.; Amaro, A.; Barra, C.; Silva, D.; Oliveira, S.; Seica, R.; Matafome, P. Distinct Impact of Natural Sugars from Fruit Juices and Added Sugars on Caloric Intake, Body Weight, Glycaemia, Oxidative Stress and Glycation in Diabetic Rats. *Nutrients* **2021**, *13*, 2956. [CrossRef] [PubMed]

11. Paglia, L. The sweet danger of added sugars. *Eur. J. Paediatr. Dent.* **2019**, *20*, 89. [CrossRef]
12. Schiano, C.; Grimaldi, V.; Scognamiglio, M.; Costa, D.; Soricelli, A.; Nicoletti, G.F.; Napoli, C. Soft drinks and sweeteners intake: Possible contribution to the development of metabolic syndrome and cardiovascular diseases. Beneficial or detrimental action of alternative sweeteners? *Food Res. Int.* **2021**, *142*, 110220. [CrossRef]
13. Te Morenga, L.; Mallard, S.; Mann, J. Dietary sugars and body weight: Systematic review and meta-analyses of randomised controlled trials and cohort studies. *BMJ* **2012**, *346*, e7492. [CrossRef] [PubMed]
14. Fan, X.; Jin, Y.; Chen, G.; Ma, X.; Zhang, L. Gut Microbiota Dysbiosis Drives the Development of Colorectal Cancer. *Digestion* **2021**, *102*, 508–515. [CrossRef] [PubMed]
15. Nikolova, V.L.; Hall, M.R.B.; Hall, L.J.; Cleare, A.J.; Stone, J.M.; Young, A.H. Perturbations in Gut Microbiota Composition in Psychiatric Disorders: A Review and Meta-analysis. *JAMA Psychiatry* **2021**, *78*, 1343–1354. [CrossRef] [PubMed]
16. Zhong, W.; Zhou, Z. Alterations of the gut microbiome and metabolome in alcoholic liver disease. *World J. Gastrointest. Pathophysiol.* **2014**, *5*, 514–522. [CrossRef] [PubMed]
17. Yang, T.; Santisteban, M.M.; Rodriguez, V.; Li, E.; Ahmari, N.; Carvajal, J.M.; Zadeh, M.; Gong, M.; Qi, Y.; Zubcevic, J.; et al. Gut dysbiosis is linked to hypertension. *Hypertension* **2015**, *65*, 1331–1340. [CrossRef] [PubMed]
18. Del Pozo, S.; Gomez-Martinez, S.; Diaz, L.E.; Nova, E.; Urrialde, R.; Marcos, A. Potential Effects of Sucralose and Saccharin on Gut Microbiota: A Review. *Nutrients* **2022**, *14*, 1682. [CrossRef]
19. Rinninella, E.; Cintoni, M.; Raoul, P.; Lopetuso, L.R.; Scaldaferri, F.; Pulcini, G.; Miggiano, G.A.D.; Gasbarrini, A.; Mele, M.C. Food Components and Dietary Habits: Keys for a Healthy Gut Microbiota Composition. *Nutrients* **2019**, *11*, 2393. [CrossRef]
20. Satokari, R. High Intake of Sugar and the Balance between Pro- and Anti-Inflammatory Gut Bacteria. *Nutrients* **2020**, *12*, 1348. [CrossRef]
21. Adithya, K.K.; Rajeev, R.; Selvin, J.; Seghal Kiran, G. Dietary Influence on the Dynamics of the Human Gut Microbiome: Prospective Implications in Interventional Therapies. *ACS Food Sci. Technol.* **2021**, *1*, 717–736. [CrossRef]
22. Freeman, C.R.; Zehra, A.; Ramirez, V.; Wiers, C.E.; Volkow, N.D.; Wang, G.J. Impact of sugar on the body, brain, and behavior. *Front. Biosci.* **2018**, *23*, 2255–2266. [CrossRef]
23. Shi, Y.N.; Liu, Y.J.; Xie, Z.; Zhang, W.J. Fructose and metabolic diseases: Too much to be good. *Chin. Med. J.* **2021**, *134*, 1276–1285. [CrossRef] [PubMed]
24. Softic, S.; Stanhope, K.L.; Boucher, J.; Divanovic, S.; Lanaspa, M.A.; Johnson, R.J.; Kahn, C.R. Fructose and hepatic insulin resistance. *Crit. Rev. Clin. Lab. Sci.* **2020**, *57*, 308–322. [CrossRef] [PubMed]
25. Fernandes, R.; Viana, S.D.; Nunes, S.; Reis, F. Diabetic gut microbiota dysbiosis as an inflammaging and immunosenescence condition that fosters progression of retinopathy and nephropathy. *Biochim. Biophys. Acta (BBA)—Mol. Basis Dis.* **2019**, *1865*, 1876–1897. [CrossRef] [PubMed]
26. Viana, S.D.; Nunes, S.; Reis, F. ACE2 imbalance as a key player for the poor outcomes in COVID-19 patients with age-related comorbidities—Role of gut microbiota dysbiosis. *Ageing Res. Rev.* **2020**, *62*, 101123. [CrossRef] [PubMed]
27. Bergeron, A.; Labonte, M.E.; Brassard, D.; Bedard, A.; Laramee, C.; Robitaille, J.; Desroches, S.; Provencher, V.; Couillard, C.; Vohl, M.C.; et al. Intakes of Total, Free, and Naturally Occurring Sugars in the French-Speaking Adult Population of the Province of Quebec, Canada: The PREDISE Study. *Nutrients* **2019**, *11*, 2317. [CrossRef] [PubMed]
28. van Loveren, C. Sugar Restriction for Caries Prevention: Amount and Frequency. Which Is More Important? *Caries Res.* **2019**, *53*, 168–175. [CrossRef]
29. World Health Organization. *WHO Guideline: Sugars Intake for Adults and Children*; World Health Organization: Geneva, Switzerland, 2015.
30. Fidler Mis, N.; Braegger, C.; Bronsky, J.; Campoy, C.; Domellof, M.; Embleton, N.D.; Hojsak, I.; Hulst, J.; Indrio, F.; Lapillonne, A.; et al. Sugar in Infants, Children and Adolescents: A Position Paper of the European Society for Paediatric Gastroenterology, Hepatology and Nutrition Committee on Nutrition. *J. Pediatr. Gastroenterol. Nutr.* **2017**, *65*, 681–696. [CrossRef]
31. Johnson, R.K.; Appel, L.J.; Brands, M.; Howard, B.V.; Lefevre, M.; Lustig, R.H.; Sacks, F.; Steffen, L.M., Wylie Rosett, J.; American Heart Association Nutrition Committee of the Council on Nutrition, Physical Activity, and Metabolism and the Council on Epidemiology and Prevention. Dietary sugars intake and cardiovascular health: A scientific statement from the American Heart Association. *Circulation* **2009**, *120*, 1011–1020. [CrossRef]
32. Plaza-Diaz, J.; Gil, A. Sucrose: Dietary Importance. In *Encyclopedia of Food and Health*; Caballero, B., Finglas, P.M., Toldrá, F., Eds.; Academic Press: Oxford, UK, 2016; pp. 199–204. [CrossRef]
33. Amarra, M.S.; Khor, G.L.; Chan, P. Intake of added sugar in Malaysia: A review. *Asia Pac. J. Clin. Nutr.* **2016**, *25*, 227–240. [CrossRef]
34. Piekara, A.; Krzywonos, M.; Szymańska, A. Sweetening Agents and Sweeteners in Dietary Supplements for Children-Analysis of the Polish Market. *Nutrients* **2020**, *12*, 2387. [CrossRef]
35. Fitch, C.; Keim, K.S. Position of the Academy of Nutrition and Dietetics: Use of nutritive and nonnutritive sweeteners. *Acad. Nutr. Diet.* **2012**, *112*, 739–758. [CrossRef] [PubMed]
36. Grembecka, M. Natural sweeteners in a human diet. *Rocz. Panstw. Zakl. Hig.* **2015**, *66*, 195–202. [PubMed]
37. MC, Y.-B. Sweeteners. In *Encyclopedia of Analytical Science*, 2nd ed.; Worsfold, P., Townshend, A., Poole, C., Eds.; Elsevier: Oxford, UK, 2005; pp. 562–572.

38. Blekas, G.A. Food Additives: Classification, Uses and Regulation. In *Encyclopedia of Food and Health*; Caballero, B., Finglas, P.M. Toldrá, F., Eds.; Academic Press: Oxford, UK, 2016; pp. 731–736. [CrossRef]
39. Hess, J.; Latulippe, M.E.; Ayoob, K.; Slavin, J. The confusing world of dietary sugars: Definitions, intakes, food sources and international dietary recommendations. *Food Funct.* **2012**, *3*, 477–486. [CrossRef] [PubMed]
40. Das, A.K.; Chakraborty, R. Sweeteners: Classification, Sensory and Health Effects. In *Encyclopedia of Food and Health*; Academic Press: Cambridge, MA, USA, 2016. [CrossRef]
41. Lenhart, A.; Chey, W.D. A Systematic Review of the Effects of Polyols on Gastrointestinal Health and Irritable Bowel Syndrome *Adv. Nutr.* **2017**, *8*, 587–596. [CrossRef]
42. Msomi, N.Z.; Erukainure, O.L.; Islam, M.S. Suitability of sugar alcohols as antidiabetic supplements: A review. *J. Food Drug Anal* **2021**, *29*, 1–14. [CrossRef]
43. Plaza-Diaz, J.; Pastor-Villaescusa, B.; Rueda-Robles, A.; Abadia-Molina, F.; Ruiz-Ojeda, F.J. Plausible Biological Interactions of Low- and Non-Calorie Sweeteners with the Intestinal Microbiota: An Update of Recent Studies. *Nutrients* **2020**, *12*, 1153 [CrossRef]
44. Carocho, M.; Morales, P.; Ferreira, I. Sweeteners as food additives in the XXI century: A review of what is known, and what is to come. *Food Chem. Toxicol.* **2017**, *107*, 302–317. [CrossRef]
45. Ruiz-Ojeda, F.J.; Plaza-Diaz, J.; Saez-Lara, M.J.; Gil, A. Effects of Sweeteners on the Gut Microbiota: A Review of Experimental Studies and Clinical Trials. *Adv. Nutr.* **2019**, *10*, S31–S48. [CrossRef]
46. Chaturvedula, V.S.; Upreti, M.; Prakash, I. Diterpene glycosides from Stevia rebaudiana. *Molecules* **2011**, *16*, 3552–3562. [CrossRef]
47. Baker-Smith, C.M.; de Ferranti, S.D.; Cochran, W.J.; Abrams, S.A.; Fuchs, G.J.; Kim, J.H.; Lindsey, C.W.; Magge, S.N.; Rome, E.S.; Schwarzenberg, S.J.; et al. The Use of Nonnutritive Sweeteners in Children. *Pediatrics* **2019**, *144*, e20192765. [CrossRef]
48. Walbolt, J.; Koh, Y. Non-nutritive Sweeteners and Their Associations with Obesity and Type 2 Diabetes. *J. Obes. Metab. Syndr.* **2020**, *29*, 114–123. [CrossRef] [PubMed]
49. Liu, X. Microbiome. *Yale J. Biol. Med.* **2016**, *89*, 275–276.
50. Cunningham, A.L.; Stephens, J.W.; Harris, D.A. Intestinal microbiota and their metabolic contribution to type 2 diabetes and obesity. *J. Diabetes Metab. Disord.* **2021**, *20*, 1855–1870. [CrossRef] [PubMed]
51. Turnbaugh, P.J.; Ley, R.E.; Hamady, M.; Fraser-Liggett, C.M.; Knight, R.; Gordon, J.I. The human microbiome project. *Nature* **2007**, *449*, 804–810. [CrossRef] [PubMed]
52. Bull, M.J.; Plummer, N.T. Part 1: The Human Gut Microbiome in Health and Disease. *Integr. Med.* **2014**, *13*, 17–22.
53. Borse, S.P.; Chhipa, A.S.; Sharma, V.; Singh, D.P.; Nivsarkar, M. Management of Type 2 Diabetes: Current Strategies, Unfocussed Aspects, Challenges, and Alternatives. *Med. Princ. Pract.* **2021**, *30*, 109–121. [CrossRef] [PubMed]
54. Doumatey, A.P.; Adeyemo, A.; Zhou, J.; Lei, L.; Adebamowo, S.N.; Adebamowo, C.; Rotimi, C.N. Gut Microbiome Profiles Are Associated With Type 2 Diabetes in Urban Africans. *Front. Cell Infect. Microbiol.* **2020**, *10*, 63. [CrossRef]
55. Larsen, N.; Vogensen, F.K.; van den Berg, F.W.; Nielsen, D.S.; Andreasen, A.S.; Pedersen, B.K.; Al-Soud, W.A.; Sorensen, S.J.; Hansen, L.H.; Jakobsen, M. Gut microbiota in human adults with type 2 diabetes differs from non-diabetic adults. *PLoS ONE* **2010**, *5*, e9085. [CrossRef] [PubMed]
56. Silva, Y.P.; Bernardi, A.; Frozza, R.L. The Role of Short-Chain Fatty Acids From Gut Microbiota in Gut-Brain Communication. *Front. Endocrinol* **2020**, *11*, 25. [CrossRef]
57. den Besten, G.; van Eunen, K.; Groen, A.K.; Venema, K.; Reijngoud, D.J.; Bakker, B.M. The role of short-chain fatty acids in the interplay between diet, gut microbiota, and host energy metabolism. *J. Lipid Res.* **2013**, *54*, 2325–2340. [CrossRef]
58. He, J.; Zhang, P.; Shen, L.; Niu, L.; Tan, Y.; Chen, L.; Zhao, Y.; Bai, L.; Hao, X.; Li, X.; et al. Short-Chain Fatty Acids and Their Association with Signalling Pathways in Inflammation, Glucose and Lipid Metabolism. *Int. J. Mol. Sci.* **2020**, *21*, 6356. [CrossRef] [PubMed]
59. Peng, L.; Li, Z.R.; Green, R.S.; Holzman, I.R.; Lin, J. Butyrate enhances the intestinal barrier by facilitating tight junction assembly via activation of AMP-activated protein kinase in Caco-2 cell monolayers. *J. Nutr.* **2009**, *139*, 1619–1625. [CrossRef] [PubMed]
60. Priyadarshini, M.; Kotlo, K.U.; Dudeja, P.K.; Layden, B.T. Role of Short Chain Fatty Acid Receptors in Intestinal Physiology and Pathophysiology. *Compr. Physiol.* **2018**, *8*, 1091–1115. [CrossRef] [PubMed]
61. Correa-Oliveira, R.; Fachi, J.L.; Vieira, A.; Sato, F.T.; Vinolo, M.A. Regulation of immune cell function by short-chain fatty acids. *Clin. Transl. Immunol.* **2016**, *5*, e73. [CrossRef] [PubMed]
62. Carretta, M.D.; Quiroga, J.; Lopez, R.; Hidalgo, M.A.; Burgos, R.A. Participation of Short-Chain Fatty Acids and Their Receptors in Gut Inflammation and Colon Cancer. *Front. Physiol.* **2021**, *12*, 662739. [CrossRef] [PubMed]
63. Brown, A.J.; Goldsworthy, S.M.; Barnes, A.A.; Eilert, M.M.; Tcheang, L.; Daniels, D.; Muir, A.I.; Wigglesworth, M.J.; Kinghorn, I.; Fraser, N.J.; et al. The Orphan G protein-coupled receptors GPR41 and GPR43 are activated by propionate and other short chain carboxylic acids. *J. Biol. Chem.* **2003**, *278*, 11312–11319. [CrossRef] [PubMed]
64. Park, J.; Wang, Q.; Wu, Q.; Mao-Draayer, Y.; Kim, C.H. Author Correction: Bidirectional regulatory potentials of short-chain fatty acids and their G-protein-coupled receptors in autoimmune neuroinflammation. *Sci. Rep.* **2019**, *9*, 17511. [CrossRef] [PubMed]
65. Layden, B.T.; Angueira, A.R.; Brodsky, M.; Durai, V.; Lowe, W.L. Short chain fatty acids and their receptors: New metabolic targets. *Transl. Res.* **2013**, *161*, 131–140. [CrossRef] [PubMed]
66. Larraufie, P.; Martin-Gallausiaux, C.; Lapaque, N.; Dore, J.; Gribble, F.M.; Reimann, F.; Blottiere, H.M. SCFAs strongly stimulate PYY production in human enteroendocrine cells. *Sci. Rep.* **2018**, *8*, 74. [CrossRef] [PubMed]

67. Tazoe, H.; Otomo, Y.; Kaji, I.; Tanaka, R.; Karaki, S.I.; Kuwahara, A. Roles of short-chain fatty acids receptors, GPR41 and GPR43 on colonic functions. *J. Physiol. Pharmacol.* **2008**, *59* (Suppl. S2), 251–262. [PubMed]
68. Hernandez, M.A.G.; Canfora, E.E.; Jocken, J.W.E.; Blaak, E.E. The Short-Chain Fatty Acid Acetate in Body Weight Control and Insulin Sensitivity. *Nutrients* **2019**, *11*, 1943. [CrossRef]
69. Martin-Gallausiaux, C.; Marinelli, L.; Blottiere, H.M.; Larraufie, P.; Lapaque, N. SCFA: Mechanisms and functional importance in the gut. *Proc. Nutr. Soc.* **2021**, *80*, 37–49. [CrossRef] [PubMed]
70. Perry, R.J.; Peng, L.; Barry, N.A.; Cline, G.W.; Zhang, D.; Cardone, R.L.; Petersen, K.F.; Kibbey, R.G.; Goodman, A.L.; Shulman, G.I. Acetate mediates a microbiome-brain-beta-cell axis to promote metabolic syndrome. *Nature* **2016**, *534*, 213–217. [CrossRef] [PubMed]
71. Trent, C.M.; Blaser, M.J. Microbially Produced Acetate: A "Missing Link" in Understanding Obesity? *Cell Metab.* **2016**, *24*, 9–10. [CrossRef] [PubMed]
72. Hamer, H.M.; Jonkers, D.; Venema, K.; Vanhoutvin, S.; Troost, F.J.; Brummer, R.J. Review article: The role of butyrate on colonic function. *Aliment. Pharmacol. Ther.* **2008**, *27*, 104–119. [CrossRef]
73. Ji, J.; Shu, D.; Zheng, M.; Wang, J.; Luo, C.; Wang, Y.; Guo, F.; Zou, X.; Lv, X.; Li, Y.; et al. Microbial metabolite butyrate facilitates M2 macrophage polarization and function. *Sci. Rep.* **2016**, *6*, 24838. [CrossRef]
74. Leonardini, A.; Laviola, L.; Perrini, S.; Natalicchio, A.; Giorgino, F. Cross-Talk between PPARgamma and Insulin Signaling and Modulation of Insulin Sensitivity. *PPAR Res.* **2009**, *2009*, 818945. [CrossRef] [PubMed]
75. Wang, D.; Shi, L.; Xin, W.; Xu, J.; Xu, J.; Li, Q.; Xu, Z.; Wang, J.; Wang, G.; Yao, W.; et al. Activation of PPARgamma inhibits pro-inflammatory cytokines production by upregulation of miR-124 in vitro and in vivo. *Biochem. Biophys. Res. Commun.* **2017**, *486*, 726–731. [CrossRef] [PubMed]
76. Peng, L.; He, Z.; Chen, W.; Holzman, I.R.; Lin, J. Effects of butyrate on intestinal barrier function in a Caco-2 cell monolayer model of intestinal barrier. *Pediatr. Res.* **2007**, *61*, 37–41. [CrossRef] [PubMed]
77. De Vadder, F.; Kovatcheva-Datchary, P.; Goncalves, D.; Vinera, J.; Zitoun, C.; Duchampt, A.; Backhed, F.; Mithieux, G. Microbiota-generated metabolites promote metabolic benefits via gut-brain neural circuits. *Cell* **2014**, *156*, 84–96. [CrossRef] [PubMed]
78. Feuerer, M.; Herrero, L.; Cipolletta, D.; Naaz, A.; Wong, J.; Nayer, A.; Lee, J.; Goldfine, A.B.; Benoist, C.; Shoelson, S.; et al. Lean, but not obese, fat is enriched for a unique population of regulatory T cells that affect metabolic parameters. *Nat. Med.* **2009**, *15*, 930–939. [CrossRef] [PubMed]
79. Shimizu, J.; Kubota, T.; Takada, E.; Takai, K.; Fujiwara, N.; Arimitsu, N.; Murayama, M.A.; Ueda, Y.; Wakisaka, S.; Suzuki, T.; et al. Propionate-producing bacteria in the intestine may associate with skewed responses of IL10-producing regulatory T cells in patients with relapsing polychondritis. *PLoS ONE* **2018**, *13*, e0203657. [CrossRef] [PubMed]
80. Ludwig, D.S.; Hu, F.B.; Tappy, L.; Brand-Miller, J. Dietary carbohydrates: Role of quality and quantity in chronic disease. *BMJ* **2018**, *361*, k2340. [CrossRef]
81. Seo, Y.S.; Lee, H.B.; Kim, Y.; Park, H.Y. Dietary Carbohydrate Constituents Related to Gut Dysbiosis and Health. *Microorganisms* **2020**, *8*, 427. [CrossRef] [PubMed]
82. Goodman, B.E. Insights into digestion and absorption of major nutrients in humans. *Adv. Physiol. Educ.* **2010**, *34*, 44–53. [CrossRef] [PubMed]
83. Do, M.H.; Lee, E.; Oh, M.-J.; Kim, Y.; Park, H.-Y. High-Glucose or -Fructose Diet Cause Changes of the Gut Microbiota and Metabolic Disorders in Mice without Body Weight Change. *Nutrients* **2018**, *10*, 761. [CrossRef]
84. Wang, Y.; Qi, W.; Song, G.; Pang, S.; Peng, Z.; Li, Y.; Wang, P. High-Fructose Diet Increases Inflammatory Cytokines and Alters Gut Microbiota Composition in Rats. *Mediat. Inflamm.* **2020**, *2020*, 6672636. [CrossRef] [PubMed]
85. Sun, S.; Araki, Y.; Hanzawa, F.; Umeki, M.; Kojima, T.; Nishimura, N.; Ikeda, S.; Mochizuki, S.; Oda, H. High sucrose diet-induced dysbiosis of gut microbiota promotes fatty liver and hyperlipidemia in rats. *J. Nutr. Biochem.* **2021**, *93*, 108621. [CrossRef] [PubMed]
86. Xiang, S.; Ye, K.; Li, M.; Ying, J.; Wang, H.; Han, J.; Shi, L.; Xiao, J.; Shen, Y.; Feng, X.; et al. Xylitol enhances synthesis of propionate in the colon via cross-feeding of gut microbiota. *Microbiome* **2021**, *9*, 62. [CrossRef] [PubMed]
87. Zuo, Q.-L.; Cai, X.; Zheng, X.-Y.; Chen, D.-S.; Li, M.; Liu, Z.-Q.; Chen, K.-Q.; Han, F.-F.; Zhu, X. Influences of Xylitol Consumption at Different Dosages on Intestinal Tissues and Gut Microbiota in Rats. *J. Agric. Food Chem.* **2021**, *69*, 12002–12011. [CrossRef]
88. Sarmiento-Rubiano, L.A.; Zuniga, M.; Perez-Martinez, G.; Yebra, M.J. Dietary supplementation with sorbitol results in selective enrichment of lactobacilli in rat intestine. *Res. Microbiol.* **2007**, *158*, 694–701. [CrossRef] [PubMed]
89. Peuranen, S.; Tiihonen, K.; Apajalahti, J.; Kettunen, A.; Saarinen, M.; Rautonen, N. Combination of polydextrose and lactitol affects microbial ecosystem and immune responses in rat gastrointestinal tract. *Br. J. Nutr.* **2004**, *91*, 905–914. [CrossRef]
90. Uebanso, T.; Kano, S.; Yoshimoto, A.; Naito, C.; Shimohata, T.; Mawatari, K.; Takahashi, A. Effects of Consuming Xylitol on Gut Microbiota and Lipid Metabolism in Mice. *Nutrients* **2017**, *9*, 756. [CrossRef] [PubMed]
91. Amo, K.; Arai, H.; Uebanso, T.; Fukaya, M.; Koganei, M.; Sasaki, H.; Yamamoto, H.; Taketani, Y.; Takeda, E. Effects of xylitol on metabolic parameters and visceral fat accumulation. *J. Clin. Biochem. Nutr.* **2011**, *49*, 1–7. [CrossRef] [PubMed]
92. Suez, J.; Korem, T.; Zeevi, D.; Zilberman-Schapira, G.; Thaiss, C.A.; Maza, O.; Israeli, D.; Zmora, N.; Gilad, S.; Weinberger, A.; et al. Artificial sweeteners induce glucose intolerance by altering the gut microbiota. *Nature* **2014**, *514*, 181–186. [CrossRef] [PubMed]
93. Bian, X.; Tu, P.; Chi, L.; Gao, B.; Ru, H.; Lu, K. Saccharin induced liver inflammation in mice by altering the gut microbiota and its metabolic functions. *Food Chem. Toxicol.* **2017**, *107 Pt B*, 530–539. [CrossRef]

94. Daly, K.; Darby, A.C.; Hall, N.; Nau, A.; Bravo, D.; Shirazi-Beechey, S.P. Dietary supplementation with lactose or artificial sweetener enhances swine gut Lactobacillus population abundance. *Br. J. Nutr.* **2014**, *111* (Suppl. S1), S30–S35. [CrossRef]
95. Abou-Donia, M.B.; El-Masry, E.M.; Abdel-Rahman, A.A.; McLendon, R.E.; Schiffman, S.S. Splenda alters gut microflora and increases intestinal p-glycoprotein and cytochrome p-450 in male rats. *J. Toxicol. Environ. Health A* **2008**, *71*, 1415–1429. [CrossRef] [PubMed]
96. Uebanso, T.; Ohnishi, A.; Kitayama, R.; Yoshimoto, A.; Nakahashi, M.; Shimohata, T.; Mawatari, K.; Takahashi, A. Effects of Low-Dose Non-Caloric Sweetener Consumption on Gut Microbiota in Mice. *Nutrients* **2017**, *9*, 560. [CrossRef] [PubMed]
97. Bian, X.; Chi, L.; Gao, B.; Tu, P.; Ru, H.; Lu, K. The artificial sweetener acesulfame potassium affects the gut microbiome and body weight gain in CD-1 mice. *PLoS ONE* **2017**, *12*, e0178426. [CrossRef]
98. De la Garza, A.L.; Romero-Delgado, B.; Martinez-Tamez, A.M.; Cardenas-Tueme, M.; Camacho-Zamora, B.D.; Matta-Yee-Chig, D.; Sanchez-Tapia, M.; Torres, N.; Camacho-Morales, A. Maternal Sweeteners Intake Modulates Gut Microbiota and Exacerbates Learning and Memory Processes in Adult Male Offspring. *Front. Pediatr.* **2021**, *9*, 746437. [CrossRef]
99. Palmnas, M.S.; Cowan, T.E.; Bomhof, M.R.; Su, J.; Reimer, R.A.; Vogel, H.J.; Hittel, D.S.; Shearer, J. Low-dose aspartame consumption differentially affects gut microbiota-host metabolic interactions in the diet-induced obese rat. *PLoS ONE* **2014**, *9*, e109841. [CrossRef]
100. Lu, J.F.; Zhu, M.Q.; Zhang, H.; Liu, H.; Xia, B.; Wang, Y.L.; Shi, X.; Peng, L.; Wu, J.W. Neohesperidin attenuates obesity by altering the composition of the gut microbiota in high-fat diet-fed mice. *FASEB J.* **2020**, *34*, 12053–12071. [CrossRef]
101. Chi, L.; Bian, X.; Gao, B.; Tu, P.; Lai, Y.; Ru, H.; Lu, K. Effects of the Artificial Sweetener Neotame on the Gut Microbiome and Fecal Metabolites in Mice. *Molecules* **2018**, *23*, 367. [CrossRef]
102. Li, X.Y.; He, C.; Zhu, Y.; Lu, N.H. Role of gut microbiota on intestinal barrier function in acute pancreatitis. *World J. Gastroenterol.* **2020**, *26*, 2187–2193. [CrossRef]
103. Verhaar, B.J.H.; Prodan, A.; Nieuwdorp, M.; Muller, M. Gut Microbiota in Hypertension and Atherosclerosis: A Review. *Nutrients* **2020**, *12*, 2982. [CrossRef]
104. Zaky, A.; Glastras, S.J.; Wong, M.Y.W.; Pollock, C.A.; Saad, S. The Role of the Gut Microbiome in Diabetes and Obesity-Related Kidney Disease. *Int. J. Mol. Sci.* **2021**, *22*, 9641. [CrossRef]
105. Gardner, C.; Wylie-Rosett, J.; Gidding, S.S.; Steffen, L.M.; Johnson, R.K.; Reader, D.; Lichtenstein, A.H.; American Heart Association Nutrition Committee of the Council on Nutrition, Physical Activity and Metabolism, Council on Arteriosclerosis, Thrombosis and Vascular Biology, Council on Cardiovascular Disease in the Young, and the American Diabetes Association. Nonnutritive sweeteners: Current use and health perspectives: A scientific statement from the American Heart Association and the American Diabetes Association. *Diabetes Care* **2012**, *35*, 1798–1808. [CrossRef]
106. Narayanan, S.; Bhutiani, N.; Adamson, D.T.; Jones, C.M. Pancreatectomy, Islet Cell Transplantation, and Nutrition Considerations. *Nutr. Clin. Pract.* **2021**, *36*, 385–397. [CrossRef]

diabetology

MDPI

Review

Are Dietary Sugars Potent Adipose Tissue and Immune Cell Modulators?

Pedro Barbosa [1,2,3] and Eugenia Carvalho [2,3,*]

1 PhD Programme in Experimental Biology and Biomedicine, Institute for Interdisciplinary Research, University of Coimbra, 3030-789 Coimbra, Portugal
2 Institute for Interdisciplinary Research, University of Coimbra, 3030-789 Coimbra, Portugal
3 Center for Neuroscience and Cell Biology, University of Coimbra, 3004-504 Coimbra, Portugal
* Correspondence: ecarvalh@cnc.uc.pt

Abstract: Glucose, fructose, and galactose are widely used in the food industry as sweeteners and food additives. The over-consumption of these carbohydrates has been identified as a possible trigger of non-communicable diseases. These include insulin resistance, obesity, and type 2 diabetes. These sugars induce an energy overload with consequent adipose tissue (AT) expansion, contributing to the development of obesity. Furthermore, a common feature of these non-communicable diseases is the detrimental, chronic, low-grade inflammation contributing to their onset. In the present review, we identify the most widely used dietary free sugars and their direct impacts on AT metabolism and inflammation, as well as their involvement in systemic inflammation and effects on the immune cell phenotype and function. Additionally, we discuss the capacity of the free sugars to induce immune modulation, enhancing inflammation, an underlying hallmark of insulin resistance, obesity, and T2DM. Dietary sugars have an important and deleterious metabolic impact on AT and also on immune cells. More research is needed to effectively understand the impact of chronic exposure to high levels of individual or combined sugars on metabolism, with the impact on immunomodulation being especially important.

Keywords: immunomodulation; inflammation; insulin resistance; sugar metabolism; adipose tissue

Citation: Barbosa, P.; Carvalho, E. Are Dietary Sugars Potent Adipose Tissue and Immune Cell Modulators? *Diabetology* **2023**, *4*, 30–45. https://doi.org/10.3390/diabetology4010005

Academic Editor: Paulo Matafome

Received: 8 November 2022
Revised: 12 January 2023
Accepted: 14 January 2023
Published: 19 January 2023

1. Introduction

The Western diet is characterized by the presence of highly processed foods, which are particularly rich in salt, saturated fats, poor-quality protein, and simple carbohydrates, such as those deriving from corn, refined cereals, and sugars (glucose, fructose, and sucrose) [1]. Many of these carbohydrates present high glycemic and high insulinemic indices that quickly induce glucose and insulin stimulation peaks for short periods of time [2]. In contrast, diets with large contents of high-quality protein and plant-based foods, such as vegetables, nuts, fruits, and honey, which contain carbohydrates with low glycemic and low insulinemic indices, are generally considered healthier [1]. The energy overload caused by the increased consumption of refined sugars (free sugar) and saturated fats can lead to a drastic expansion of adipose tissue (AT) depots, especially when associated with a lack of physical activity [3]. In addition, a reduction in the fiber content of ingested foods may support metabolic destabilization, since sugars are quickly and freely available in the system [4,5]. Therefore, the Western diet has been identified as a possible trigger of the development of non-communicable diseases from an early stage of life. Insulin resistance (IR), obesity, type 2 diabetes mellitus (T2DM), and metabolic syndrome are some of the most prevalent non-communicable diseases worldwide [1,6,7].

In the present review, we discuss the most widely used dietary sugars and their impacts on metabolism, systemic inflammation, and AT-specific inflammation. Furthermore, we discuss how these sugars are capable of modulating the immune cells and their immunometabolism, promoting inflammation, an underlying hallmark of insulin resistance, obesity, and T2DM.

2. Dietary (Free) Sugars

Free sugars are mono- and disaccharides that are added to food, excluding the naturally present types, such as lactose in milk and sucrose in fruits and vegetables, although these naturally present sugars can be considered as free sugars when they are added to a product (Figure 1) [3,8]. Generally, free sugars are widely used in the food industry as sweeteners and food additives, especially in beverages and during food transformation and preparation [3,8], appearing in large proportions in the Western diet [9]. The monosaccharides, glucose, and fructose, as well as disaccharides, sucrose, and lactose, are used as additives in the Western diet [3,10], with fructose and glucose representing almost 50% of the added sugars [11]. These two monosaccharides are commonly used individually or in the form of sucrose or high-fructose corn syrup (HFCS). Sucrose is extracted and purified from sugar cane and sugar beet, while fructose is obtained by the enzymatic degradation of cornstarch into glucose or glucose polymers to be further isomerized enzymatically into fructose, producing the HFCS [3]. The main difference between sucrose and HFCS lies in the fructose content, which varies between 42% and 55% in HFCS and is 50% in sucrose. Moreover, sucrose is composed of glucose covalently bonded to fructose, while in HFCS, these molecules remain in their free forms, rendering them highly bioavailable and increasing their absorption when consumed [3,12]. Lactose is also widely used not only in the food industry, where it is applied in the form of condensed milk and in caramel flavors, but also in the pharmaceutical industry as a drug carrier [13]. In similarity to sucrose, lactose is a disaccharide of glucose and galactose that is used frequently in the confectionery and bakery industries. The production of caramel flavors using lactose depends on the Maillard reaction [13]. In the bakery industry, this process is important for creating the brown color of products, since lactose is not degraded by yeast [13].

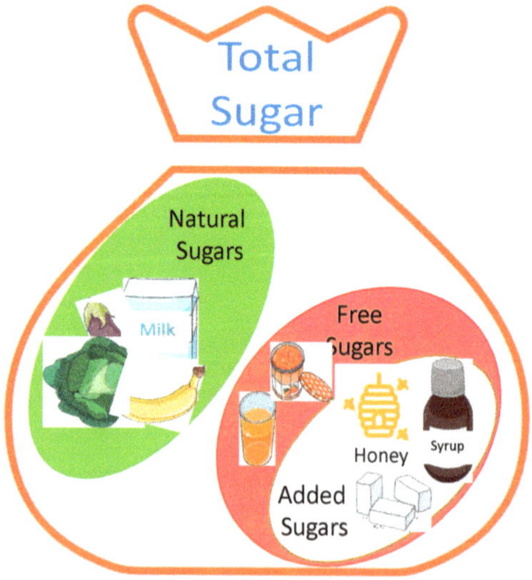

Figure 1. Total sugar content of a product: The total sugar of a product consists of its natural sugar content and/or the sugar added during its preparation, although, in some cases, natural sugars can be considered as free sugars, since they are easily bioavailable. Additionally, honey can be used as an added sugar in the food industry. The figure was created using pictures from Servier Medical Art (smart.servier.com). Servier Medical Art by Servier is licensed under a Creative Commons Attribution 3.0 Unported License (https://creativecommons.org/licenses/by/3.0/, accessed on 27 October 2022).

3. Sugar Metabolism and Its Effect on Adipose Tissue

In different proportions, all the sugars described above are widely used in the Western diet, and there is no consensus regarding their potential harmful effects on metabolism [11,14]. Sucrose and HFCS are composed of monomers of fructose and glucose, and despite their similar structures, they follow different metabolic pathways, as described below [15], while galactose, resulting from lactose, follows the Leloir metabolic pathway [16] (Figure 2).

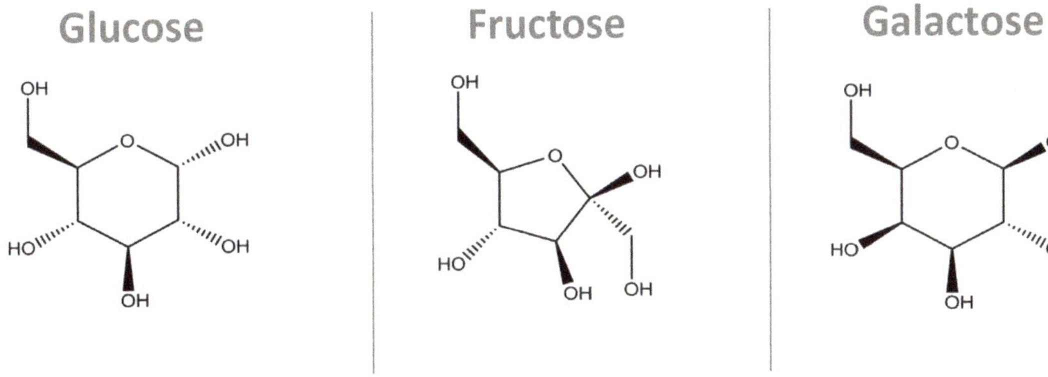

Figure 2. Molecular structure of the main monosaccharides that compose our diet. Despite their similarity in terms of the molecular structures, their conformations are different, causing them to interact with their microenvironments in different ways. Additionally, their metabolic pathways are different. These three molecules are the carbon skeleton for sucrose (glucose + fructose bonded by a α1,β2-glycosidic bond) and for lactose (glucose + galactose bonded by a β1,4-glycosidic bond) [17].

3.1. Sucrose and HFCS—Fructose and Glucose Metabolism

After ingestion, fructose is passively absorbed by the intestinal apical membrane via the high-affinity transporter glucose transporter (GLUT)5, passed on to the portal circulation by GLUT2. On the other hand, glucose is absorbed by enterocytes, mainly through the co-transporters sodium-glucose linked transporter 1 (SGLT1) and GLUT2. Once in circulation, fructose is metabolized in the tissues by phosphofructokinase and glucokinase, and the latter is also regulated by insulin [9,15,18]. An increase in fructose consumption, associated with an unrestricted pathway, leads to a rapid increase in uric acid synthesis, gluconeogenesis, glycolysis, and de novo lipogenesis [15,19]. Unlike glucose, fructose is not regulated by the activity of phosphofructokinase, an enzyme that limits the glycolytic flux [19]. The hexo-phosphate and trios-phosphate intermediaries, resulting from fructolysis, are used as substrate for the pathways described above [15,19]. Moreover, excessive amounts of fructose will overload the liver's capacity to oxidize it. Therefore, the fructose remains in circulation and can be used by other tissues, such as AT [20]. Fructose has been described as a potential lipogenic and adipogenic nutrient accelerating lipid deposition, particularly in visceral AT, and ectopic fat deposition in the other insulin-sensitive tissues, such as the liver and muscle [19–21]. In addition, fructose has been observed to disrupt insulin sensitivity in adults [21]. Stanhope and colleagues conducted a clinical study with 32 participants aged from 40 to 72 years. The subjects were divided into two groups, including glucose- and fructose-sweetened beverage consumers, for a period of 10 weeks. The study indicated an increase in the plasma lipids and lipoproteins in the fructose consumer group, while the glucose consumer group remained unchanged, except for the triglycerides, which showed an opposite pattern. Furthermore, the authors observed alterations in insulin sensitivity and glucose tolerance after 9 weeks of beverage consumption. The fructose consumer group showed increased insulin and glucose levels during an oral glucose tolerance test compared to baseline, while the glucose consumer group remained unchanged. Moreover, the insulin sensitivity index decreased by approximately

17% in the fructose consumption group [21]. Additionally, the same study indicated that the group who consumed fructose-sweetened beverages showed a higher expression of lipogenic genes in VAT [21].

Adipocytes lack the keto-hexokinase enzyme that converts fructose into fructose-1-phosphate. In these cells, fructose is converted to fructose-6-phosphate by hexokinase stimulating the conversion of pyruvate into acetyl-CoA, thus increasing the synthesis of fatty acids, and leading to consequent palmitate release. In this case, fructose is mostly used in anabolic pathways, in contrast to glucose [22]. Interestingly, Varma and collaborators (2015) postulated that fructose can trigger the oxidation of glucose to lactate in a dose-dependent manner while reducing the utilization of glucose in the glutamate and fatty acid synthesis pathways, using a 10% $^{13}C_2$-D-glucose trace in cultured adipocytes [23]. Furthermore, the study also indicated a reduction in glucose conversion to glycogen. Consequently, glucose is driven to the one-carbon cycle and the glycine cleavage pathway (SOG pathway) through 3-phosphoglycerate to synthesize serine and other intermediates that are important for the generation of NADPH and ATP [23,24].

A treatment with 10% fructose solution in the drinking water of rats for 24 weeks induced the upregulation of genes related to the insulin-signaling pathway, particularly phosphoinositol-3-kinase (PI3K), protein kinase-B (AKT), insulin receptor(IR)-β, insulin receptor substrate (IRS)-1, and the mammalian target of rapamycin (mTOR), but also those related to adipocyte homeostasis, such as peroxisome proliferator -activated receptor (PPAR)γ and nuclear factor erythroid-2-related factor 2 (NrF2) [25], although the authors did not find any correlation between insulin impairment and adipose tissue inflammation [25]. On the other hand, different studies have suggested that fructose-rich diets affect insulin action and AT metabolism, inducing changes in the secretory patterns of resistin, adiponectin, leptin, and specific adipokines, which, in turn, are linked to inflammation and insulin resistance [26,27]. Furthermore, it has been shown that fructose induces an increase in leptin secretion and, consequently, leptin resistance [28]. However, the mechanism determining how leptin resistance is established is not well understood. Despite its different functions in the organism, leptin has a significant impact on inflammation and the inflammatory onset, not only locally at the tissue level but also systemically, perpetuating further inflammation [25,28]. In addition, Marek et al. (2015) provided important insights into the effects of fructose on the adipocyte endoplasmic reticulum (RE) redox status in mice. Moreover, increased levels of monocyte chemoattractant protein (MCP)-1, intercellular adhesion molecule (ICAM)-1, and tumor necrosis factor (TNF)-α expression by AT have already been described in response to fructose metabolism. The expression of these genes leads to an increase in macrophage infiltration on AT [28,29] but also the release of other pro-inflammatory cytokines by the adipocytes [28]. Interestingly, this inflammatory process caused by the excessive consumption of fructose-rich foods seems to have a gender-dependent impact, particularly regarding the expression of inflammatory markers in VAT [25,30]. Considering the above, Kovačević and collaborators tested the impacts of the ingestion of 10% (*w/v*) fructose solution on female and male Wistar rats for 9 weeks and noticed that, despite the diet used, there was no impact on the glucose or insulin levels. However, the fructose-treated females showed a significant reduction in the Akt and pAkt-Ser^{473} levels in VAT and an increase in the PTP1B protein levels in comparison to the standard chow, while the male rats only showed a decreased pAkt-Ser^{473}/Akt ratio. Furthermore, the fructose-treated female showed increased levels of nuclear factor (NF)κB in VAT, followed by increased levels of TNF-α, interleukin (IL)-6, and IL-1β mRNA, as well as increased levels of F4/80, a macrophage marker. In contrast, the male fructose-treated rats showed no differences in the NFκB expression levels [30].

Data suggest that fructose-rich diets induce chronic inflammation in a dose-dependent manner [31]. Wang et al. (2020) fed six-week-old Sprague Dawley male rats with low (2.6 g/kg/day), medium (5.3 g/kg/day), and high doses (10.5 g/kg/day) of fructose for 20 weeks and identified a dose-dependent increase in the circulating levels of IL-6, TNF-α, and macrophage inflammatory protein (MIP)-2 when compared to the controls, while the opposite was observed for IL-10 in an inverse pattern. In the same study, the highest fructose dose led to an increase in the number of inflammatory cells in the pancreas, a 10% increase in liver steatosis, colon inflammation, and gut microbiota alterations. Furthermore, the acute inflammatory response to a fructose-rich diet during the postprandial state was recently studied in healthy subjects and in patients with T2DM. The data showed that the levels of IL-6 and ICAM-1 were increased in the healthy subjects in the postprandial state, while MCP-1 was increased in both the healthy subjects and in the patients with T2DM [18].

The glycemic load caused by the consumption of sucrose and HFCS has also been suggested to be a possible trigger of the inflammatory processes [32–34]. In addition, a recent study conducted by Patkar et al. (2021) indicated that the long-term (3 months) consumption of 5% (*w/v*) sucrose could be a trigger of the onset of systemic low-grade inflammation, without the induction of obesity, in male Wistar rats. Furthermore, they observed an increase in some of the immune cell populations in circulation, such as lymphocytes, basophils, and neutrophils [11].

3.2. Lactose—Galactose and Glucose

Lactose is a disaccharide composed of galactose and glucose, and it is metabolized in the intestinal lumen by lactase. A complementary mechanism of lactose metabolism is through the colonic microbiota, primarily in adults [35]. This sugar differs from the other mono- and disaccharides since it has no specific transporter to pass through the intestinal barrier. However, concentrations of around 0.02 mmol/L of lactose have already been found in circulation in healthy young adult men, contrary to what had been postulated [35]. Despite not being metabolized in other tissues, lactose seems to play a role in systemic inflammation, a topic that will be discussed further in this review. On the other hand, lactose monomers are easily metabolized by the organism.

Like fructose, galactose is absorbed by the endothelial cells, released into the blood stream, and transported to the liver via the portal vein [36]. A large amount of galactose is retained and metabolized in the liver, but small amounts remain in circulation and reach other tissues, such as AT and the skeletal muscle [36]. It follows the Leloir pathway once it enters the adipocytes [16]. Krycer et al. (2020) treated 3T3-L1 adipocytes with either 25 mM of glucose or 25 mM of galactose, and they found a reduction in lactate production by the galactose-treated cells, even after insulin stimulation [37]. On the other hand, mitochondrial respiration was increased upon treatment with galactose and upon insulin stimulation [37]. Thus, galactose appears to be used to feed a different pathway, rather than glycolysis, in the adipocytes. To test this, the authors used tracers to differentiate the galactose and glucose carbons using ^{13}C-labels (both 25 mM) [37] They found a reduction in glucose-6-phosphate after the galactose treatment [37]. The glucose-6-phosphate is considered a common point between the glucose and galactose oxidation pathways and how galactose enters the glycolytic pathway. The data indicate that galactose follows a different pathway from glycolysis and is a poor substrate for energy metabolism [16]. Interestingly, similar results were found in a study on mature adipocytes isolated from rats [37]. However, Krishna et al. (2020) did not identify any effect of 25 mM of galactose or 25 mM of lactose treatment on adipocyte differentiation [38]. Considering the low degradation rate of galactose compared to glucose, high amounts of galactose in circulation can lead to galactosemia and, consequently, to the glycation of different macromolecules, including amino acids, creating advanced glycation end products (AGEs) and reactive oxygen species (ROS) [5,39]. These molecules are responsible for tissue damage that, in turn, leads to accelerated aging [40,41]. Furthermore, studies have identified that high levels of galactose also induce an accelerated aging process, possibly due to the production of ROS and AGEs [41]. Additionally, it has been reported that both AGEs and ROS are involved in the inflammation onset through the action of the nuclear factor (NF)-κB gene [5]. On the other hand, a study conducted in cultured mammalian cells, HEK293 and HepG2, indicated that galactose induces the accumulation of fructose-6-phosphate that is necessary for the N-glycosylation process. This contributes to a reduction in starvation-induced endoplasmic reticulum stress, emphasizing the contribution of galactose to other pathways rather than energy production [42]. Interestingly, a recent study indicated that in the diet of 3-week-old postweaning mice, the substitution of glucose for galactose (1:1, mimicking lactose) instead of glucose alone for 3 weeks, prior to an HFD for 9 weeks, was enough to reduce the levels of circulating leptin when compared to glucose alone, although no differences were found in white AT leptin receptor expression, especially in the female mice [43].

Despite the widespread use of these sugars in the Western diet, more studies are required to understand the impacts of lactose and galactose on human metabolism and tissue physiology. It is crucial to elucidate their underlying physiologic mechanisms of action, especially those of tissue-specific metabolism and inflammation. Furthermore, clinical trials are necessary to observe the impacts of these sugars on the organism, since the majority of the published studies were performed in vitro or on animal models.

4. The Impact of Sugar on Immunometabolism

In addition to AT and the other insulin-sensitive organs, dietary sugars can impact metabolism in different organs, including the immune system, by affecting the function and regulatory capacity of the immune cells [11,34]. The impacts of different dietary sugars (e.g., sucrose, lactose, fructose, and glucose) on specific immune cell populations, regarding their metabolism and function, have been reported (Figure 3 and Table 1). Evidence suggests that the consumption of sucrose- or fructose-containing foods leads to an increase in the leukocytes in animal models [11,26]. A significant increase in the lymphocytes, basophils, and neutrophils was reported after the treatment of Wistar rats with 5% (*w/v*) sucrose in water for 12 weeks [11]. Similarly, Rodrigues et al. (2014) evaluated the impact of fasting with 20% sucrose- (control) and 20% fructose-containing diets on postprandial male BALB/c mice. The team showed that the sucrose- and fructose-containing diets induced an increase in the total leukocyte populations in the post-prandial state [26]. Specifically, the fructose-containing diet showed the highest impact on leukocyte proliferation, followed by an increase in the pro-inflammatory cytokines and chemokines in the liver and AT, namely IL-6, TNF-α, and CCL2, and a reduction in IL-10. This pro-inflammatory state was accompanied by an increase in neutrophil recruitment and infiltration into the liver [26]. This may have been triggered by an increase in ROS, the activity of inducible nitric oxide synthase (iNOS), and TNF-α secretion during Kuppfer cell activation, as hypothesized by Kanuri et al. (2011). Interestingly, a 30% fructose drink apparently had a stronger influence on immune cell function and activation, leading to an increase in the number of neutrophils (approx. 5.5-fold higher), as well as the expression of ICAM-1 (approx. 1.8-fold) by the neutrophils, compared to plain water after treating C57BL/6j mice for 8 weeks [44]. Other sugars, such as lactose, can also induce alterations in the immune cells leading to their immunomodulation [45,46]. Lactose is a β-galactoside that can interact with proteins, such as the galectin family, leading to changes in the microenvironment of the immune cells [46]. In particular, the binding of lactose to galactin-9 (Gal-9) reduced the engagement of Gal-9 with its receptor, T-cell immunoglobulin and mucin domain 3 (TIM-3, also known as CD366), avoiding the immune suppression of the pro-inflammatory profile of T cells [46].

The immunomodulation caused by the various dietary sugars can differ between the various immune cell populations [47]. Interestingly, immune cells are also able to change their metabolic demand, usually designated as metabolic switch. This can occur upon activation, and the carbon source that the cells use for their metabolism may influence these changes [34,48]. Usually, this metabolic switch occurs quickly upon activation, since these cells require fast ATP production to fulfill their energetic demands. Oxidative phosphorylation (OXPHOS) is reduced, while aerobic glycolysis is prioritized, in most immune cells [47,49], leading to a proinflammatory profile [48]. Menk et al. (2018) showed that the activation of naïve and memory $CD4^+$ and $CD8^+$ T cells by anti-CD3 and anti-CD28 for approximately 6 h led to an increase in glycolysis, measured by the extracellular acidification rate (ECAR), while OXPHOS was reduced, as measured by the oxygen consumption rate (OCR) [50]. Furthermore, Lee et al. (2019) studied the metabolism of classical monocytes

($CD14^+$ $CD16^-$), a subset of human monocytes, and discovered that LPS stimulation leads to an increase in the glycolysis rate of this subset of monocytes [51]. Furthermore, the authors also identified the glycolytic metabolism as a key pathway in the regulation of p38-MAPK, which is important for the activation and the adhesion function of the classical monocytes [51].

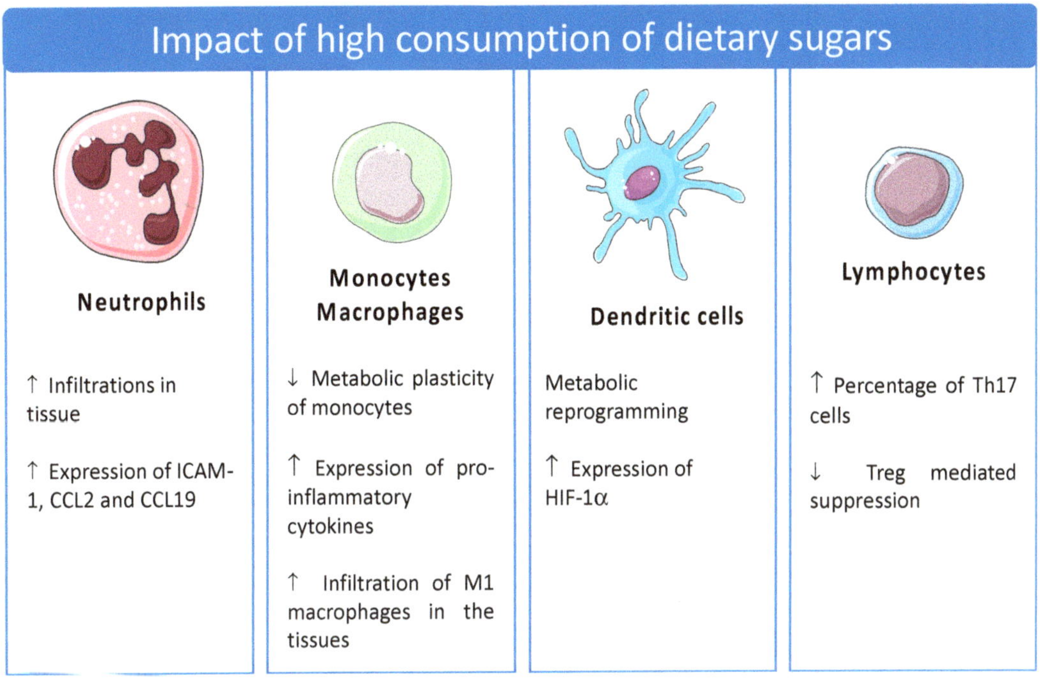

Figure 3. Effect of the excessive consumption of dietary sugars on the immune cells. The effects of dietary sugars are different in each cell type. The figure was created using pictures from Servier Medical Art (smart.servier.com). Servier Medical Art by Servier is licensed under a Creative Commons Attribution 3.0 Unported License (https://creativecommons.org/licenses/by/3.0/, accessed in 10 January 2023).

The intake of high-sugar-containing diets can enhance these important metabolic alterations, which are deleterious to human health and are some of the underlying causes of insulin resistance and T2DM development.

Table 1. Impacts of high doses of dietary sugars on immune cell populations.

Dietary Sugar	Experimental Model	Concentrations of Sugar	Treatment Duration	Impact in Immune Populations	Reference
Fructose	in vivo—IDH2 KO and C57BL/6J mice	34% fructose in H_2O	6 weeks	↑ Neutrophil infiltration into the liver of IDH2 mice	[52]
	in vivo—male C57BL/6J mice	15% fructose in H_2O	10 days	↑ Neutrophil trafficking to limbal region	[53]
	in vivo—C57BL/6J mice	30% fructose in H_2O	8 weeks	↑ Neutrophil infiltration into the liver ↑ Expression of ICAM-1, CCL2 and CCL19	[44]
	in vivo—male Swiss mice	20% fructose in H_2O	6–10 weeks	↑ Infiltration of M1 macrophages into AT ↓ Infiltration of M2 macrophages into AT	[54]
	in vitro—primary human DCs	5 to 25 mM fructose in culture medium	24–72 h	↑ Pro-inflammatory cytokine production and activation markers • Metabolic reprogramming in DCs	[34]
	in vivo—male Sprague Dawley rats	60% fructose in chow	5 weeks	↓ Immune suppressive function of Treg cells without changes in the percentage of the population	[55]
	in vitro—primary human monocytes	11.1 mM fructose in culture medium	Different time-points	↓ Metabolic plasticity of monocytes ↑ Expression of IL-1β, IL-6, IL-10, and TNF-α	[47]
	in vivo—Dahl salt-sensitive and Dahl salt-resistant rats	20% fructose in H_2O	4 weeks	↑ % of Th17 cells	[56]
Fructose and sucrose	in vivo—male BALB/c and LysM-eGFP mice	20% fructose20% sucrose (control),both in the chow	12–14 weeks	↑ Leukocyte count in circulation and infiltrated neutrophils in the liver ↓ Neutrophil infiltration into AT	[26]
Galactose	in vitro—human monocytes	11.1 mM galactose in culture medium	Different time-points	↓ Metabolic plasticity of monocytes	[47]
	in vitro—THP-1 cells	2 g/L of RPMI	5 days until experiments	↓ TNF-α expression and preference for OXPHOS	[57]
	in vitro—bone marrow DCs from male C57BL/6J mice	10 mM of galactose in culture medium	24–72 h	• Induces the maintenance of activating markers on DCs for 72h	[58]
Glucose	in vitro—human DCs	Range from 5 to 25 mM glucose in culture medium	24–72 h	↑ Expression of HIF-1α	[34]
	in vitro—human and male C57BL/6J mice CD8+ T cells	25 mM glucose	3 days	↑ Glycolysis and cytotoxic capacity of CTLs	[59]

Table 1. *Cont.*

Dietary Sugar	Experimental Model	Concentrations of Sugar	Treatment Duration	Impact in Immune Populations	Reference
Lactose	in vitro—human T cells	30 mM of lactose30 mM of sucrose in culture medium	3 days	↓ Treg immunosuppression capacity	[46]
	in vivo—female BALB/c mice	100 mg/kg of body weight	Different time-points	• Neutrophil and macrophage modulation in early acute pancreatitis • Possible interaction with lactose-Galectin 3	[45]
Sucrose	in vivo—male Wistar rats	5% (*w/v*) in H_2O	12 weeks	↑ Circulating neutrophils, lymphocytes, and basophiles	[11]
	in vivo—male Sprague Dawley	700 g/kg of chow	5 weeks	↑ $CD68^+$ macrophage infiltration into tPVAT and aPVAT ↑ Expression of MCP-1 in both tissues	[57]

↑—increase in; ↓—decrease in; IDH2 KO—isocitrate dehydrogenase 2 knock out mice; ICAM-1—intercellular adhesion molecule 1; CCL2—C-C motif chemokine ligand 2; CCL19—C-C motif chemokine ligand 19; AT—adipose tissue; DCs—dendritic cells; Treg—regulatory T cells; IL-1β—interleukin-1β; IL-6—interleukin-6; IL-10—interleukin-10; TNF-α—tumor necrosis factor-α; Th17—T helper 17 cells; OXPHOS—oxidative phosphorylation; HIF-1α—hypoxia-inducible factor-1α; CTLs—cytotoxic T lymphocytes; tPVAT—thoracic perivascular adipose tissue; aPVAT—abdominal perivascular adipose tissue; MCP-1—monocyte chemoattractant protein 1.

4.1. Monocytes/Macrophages

Macrophage infiltration may be a key mechanism leading to the pro-inflammatory status and subsequent onset of insulin resistance, especially in AT [54]. Once infiltrated into the tissues, monocytes differentiate into macrophages and usually become polarized into either pro-inflammatory M1 macrophages or anti-inflammatory M2 macrophages according to the microenvironment (Table 1). The chronic intake of a high-fructose diet (6–10 weeks; 20% fructose solution) was shown to favor the M1 macrophage subtypes, with a reduction in the number of M2 subtypes in epidydimal AT in mice. Moreover, the high recruitment of monocytes from the blood to AT ($Ly6C^+$) was observed in mice after 10 weeks on a high-fructose diet. In addition, polarization into $Ly6C^{high}$ and $Ly6C^{middle}$ M1 macrophages with a high pro-inflammatory capacity was described, with a parallel reduction in the $Ly6C^-$ M2 resident cells [54]. Jones et al. (2021) investigated the impacts of glucose (11.1 mM), fructose (11.1 mM), and galactose (11.1 mM), respectively, on the energy metabolism of circulating human monocytes. At the concentration of 11.1 mM, glucose drove the monocyte metabolism towards glycolysis, while fructose and galactose showed the opposite effect, with OXPHOS being prioritized in the basal state (Table 1). After stimulating the treated monocytes with LPS, the glucose-treated monocytes increased their glycolysis even further in contrast to the fructose- and galactose-treated monocytes, which increased in their OXPHOS capacity. However, inhibiting the hexokinase using 2-deoxyglucose, the authors noticed that the glucose-treated cells showed a reduction in ECAR followed by an increase in OCR, while the fructose- and galactose-treated monocytes indicated reductions in both ECAR and OCR [47]. Moreover, treating the fructose- and glucose-cultured monocytes with oligomycin led to a decrease in OCR in both cultures, although the fructose-treated monocytes also presented reduction in ECAR [47]. This study demonstrated the impaired metabolic flexibility in switching between OXPHOS and glycolysis for energy production by fructose, in contrast to glucose, in which case the cells can easily change their energy metabolism. Additionally, the treatment of the LPS-stimulated monocytes with fructose demonstrated a reduction in the cell viability when exposed to mitochondrial complex inhibitors, such as rotenone (complex I), antimycin A (complex III), and oligomycin (complex V), demonstrating that fructose is not a good substrate for the glycolytic pathway in human monocytes, leading to their functional impairment [47]. Furthermore, fructose had an impact in the secretory pattern of the monocytes, leading the increased secretion of IL-1β, IL-6, IL-10, and TNF-α [47]. In contrast to dendritic cells (DCs), fructose did not change the levels of surface activation marker expression in the monocytes, (e.g., HLA-DR, CD80, CD86) [47]. In addition, sucrose-enriched diets also appear to have a specific impact on macrophages, especially by increasing their proliferation in the peripheral tissues, as observed in the perivascular AT [57] and liver [60]. In accordance with the findings described by Jones et al. (2021), Millet et al. (2016) indicated that galactose (2 g/L of medium) is able to direct the monocyte metabolism towards OXPHOS, followed by a reduction in the TNF-α levels, compared to glucose at the same concentration (Table 1) [61]. Similar to galactose, the treatment of mice with lactose induced a reduction in the percentage of macrophages, but it also increased their production of IL-10 through a galectin-3–lactose interaction [45].

4.2. Dendritic Cells

Dendritic cells are important antigen-presenting cells (APCs) that allow for an adaptative immune response but also promote tolerance through the degradation of self-antigen-reactive thymocytes [34,62]. Jaiswal et al. (2019) tested concentrations ranging from 5 to 25 mM of fructose and glucose in vitro using human DCs collected from healthy donors for 24–72 h. The results indicated that 15 mM of fructose was able to induce an increase in the expression of key activation markers in the DCs, such as CD86, a co-stimulatory molecule (Table 1). This, in turn, was followed by an increase in proinflammatory cytokine secretion, including IL-1β, IL-6, and TNF-α, by the DCs. Additionally, the treatment with 15 mM of glucose also induced an increase in the expression of the TNF-α levels after 72 h.

Moreover, a co-culture of fructose-exposed DCs with $CD3^+$ T cells induced an increase in IFN-γ secretion by the T cells when compared to the control (5 mM of glucose), a possible consequence of the increased TNF-α release by the DCs when exposed to the 15 mM of fructose. Interestingly, despite the indirect effect through the DCs, the authors did not observe a direct effect of fructose on cytokine secretion in the cultured T cells. Furthermore, during the treatment of the DCs, the authors analyzed their metabolic profile, identifying a process of metabolic reprogramming through a reduction in OCR and an increase in ECAR when higher concentrations of fructose were used [34]. The reduction in OCR was supported by a reduction in the ROS production of the fructose-treated cells when compared with the glucose-treated and control DCs after 24 h of treatment [34]. After 72 h of treatment, the authors found a similar result for the fructose-treated DCs, although phospho-p70S6 kinase and hypoxia-inducible factor (HIF)-1α had higher expressions than those observed in the glucose-treated and control DCs [34]. The data suggest that cytokine secretion in fructose-treated DCs is independent of the AKT–mTOR axis [34]. The metabolic switch of the DCs culminated in their chronic activation, promoting a pro-inflammatory profile through the accumulation of advanced glycation end products, especially in the fructose-treated DCs, with the consequent enhanced activation of NF-κB [34].

On the other hand, glucose also seems to play an important role in the metabolic function of DCs and their interaction with $CD8^+$ T cells (Table 1). Lawless et al. (2017) showed that the activation of DCs with LPS for 24 h led to an increased expression of co-stimulatory molecules, such as CD80 and CD86, with a decline in their expression after 48 h and 72 h when treated with 10 mM of glucose, although, in the presence of 10 mM of galactose, the DCs maintained the expression of co-stimulatory molecules for approximately 72 h after stimulation. This co-stimulatory expression was corroborated by co-culturing the DCs with $CD8^+$ T cells for 72 h in glucose and galactose at 10 mM (Table 1). As expected, the galactose-treated DCs retained the capacity to induce the clonal expansion of the $CD8^+$ T cells for 72 h, with the further increased expression of IFNγ production by the T cells, in contrast to the glucose-treated DCs, which started to decline in their capacity to induce the $CD8^+$ T cells after 48 h of co-culture [58]. The authors also postulated that a reduction in the glucose concentration in the medium (10 mM to 2 mM) was followed by a reduction in the expression of HIF-1α in the DCs after LPS activation [58]. Interestingly, galactose was also capable of inducing a similar effect [58]. However, under 2 mM of glucose, the expression of HIF-1α was limited by the inactivation of mammalian target of rapamycin complex 1 (mTORC1) signaling, consequently inducing the activation of 5′AMP-activated protein kinase (AMPK), while under the 10 mM galactose treatment, it was enough to maintain low levels of glycolysis and OXPHOS for ATP synthesis, maintaining mTORC1 activation, and the reduction in HIF-1α was described as mTORC1-independent [58]. These data provide a good example illustrating how different dietary sugars may act in different ways, at least in vitro (Table 1). However, much research is needed in the future to understand the impacts of these sugars on more complex organisms, including the human physiology.

4.3. Lymphocytes

Lymphocytes, which comprise T, B, and NK populations, are responsible for the adaptative immune response and play important roles in tissues inflammation. In fact, T cells play an important role in AT inflammation and insulin resistance during the onset of obesity [63,64]. There are few studies that have described the impact of high-sugar diet consumption on humans (Table 1), although it has been suggested that high-sugar diets have impacts on the T cell metabolism and function [47,55]. In fact, it was demonstrated that human-activated $CD8^+$ T cells (CTLs) cultured with high glucose (25 mM, mimicking a hyperglycemic condition) led to a higher absorption of glucose, in contrast to CTLs treated with 5.6 mM of glucose, resulting in a higher glycolytic rate in the case of the high-glucose-treated CTLs [59]. Considering the importance of the glycolytic pathway in the regulation of the effector killing function of these cells, Zhu et al. (2021) postulated that a hyperglycemic microenvironment would enhance the cytotoxicity capacity of the CTLs after 3 and 6 days following in vitro activation [59]. Additionally, the authors evaluated the cytotoxic capacity of incubated CTLs from diabetic mice, compared with CTLs from healthy mice, and concluded that the CTLs collected from the diabetic mice showed a faster killing kinetic in contrast to the control [59]. However, patients with type 2 diabetes have an increased percentage of the $CCR7^{-}$ $CD45RA^{+}$ $CD8^{+}$ T cell subset compared to healthy people. This subset of $CD8^{+}$ T cells represents a decline in immune function, also called immunosenescence [65]. Furthermore, high glucose intake could be an important factor in the exacerbation of autoimmune disease, especially through the mediation of $CD4^{+}$ T helper (Th) 17 [66]. In line with this, high fructose intake (20% solution) also showed a Th17-mediated inflammation response through the production of IL-17A in Dahl salt-sensitive rats, representing a model of hypertension (Table 1) [56].

In 2013, Leibowitz et al. indicated that fructose-enriched diets, administered for 5 weeks, induced functional alterations in the T cells of Sprague Dawley rats, particularly in Treg [55]. Furthermore, after feeding the animals on a high-fructose diet (60% fructose) for 5 weeks, the authors identified the dysfunction of IL-10 production by Treg when compared to the control chow diet, even in the absence of alterations in the percentage of the Treg population [55]. On the other hand, results reported by Jaiswal et al. (2019) indicated that 15 mM of fructose did not change or have a direct effect on cultured T lymphocyte populations [34].

Lactose, in circulation, can have deleterious effects on immune cells, leading to inflammation (Table 1) [46]. Lactose has the potential to bind to *Gal-9*, reducing its ability to bind its receptor, TIM-3, on the surfaces of different immune cells, including the macrophages and T cell populations. *Gal-9*/TIM-3 signaling plays an important role in Treg cell differentiation and effector T cell exhaustion [46]. Moreover, this pathway is important for the regulation and resolution of inflammation through the regulation of the Th1 and Th17 immune responses [46]. Moreover, Paasela et al. (2014) incubated enriched Treg cells from healthy donors with effector T cells (Teff) for 3 days. They reported a decrease in IFN-γ and IL-17 secretion by Teff. However, after adding 30 mM of lactose, the authors reported a reduction in Treg-mediated suppression and a consequent increase in IFN-γ and IL-17 secretion [46]. Furthermore, the authors observed an increase in the number of $CD4^{+}$ $TIM\text{-}3^{+}$ cells producing IL-17 after incubation with lactose, even when co-cultured with Treg [46].

Naïve T lymphocytes and Treg cells preferentially utilize fatty acid substrates during their metabolism, with a low activity of mTOR. On the other hand, after activation, T cells rely mainly on aerobic glycolysis, displaying higher mTOR activity, and in the case of Treg, this can induce the downregulation of transcription factor Foxp3, promoting a reduction in the cells' proliferation [67]. Treg cells are important, as they mediate the homeostasis of the organism and counterbalance the Teff cells [67].

5. Concluding Remarks

The propagation of the Western diet has become a worldwide burden, together with the excessive consumption of free/added sugars. These can trigger chronic low-grade inflammation not only by alterations in the AT metabolism and other insulin-sensitive organs but also by the induction of critical changes in the immune system. These alterations can lead to the loss of function of important immune cell populations. Importantly, many of these alterations have key impacts on the plasticity of immune cells, reducing their capacity to adjust to the surrounding environment. However, more research needs to be performed in order to better understand the deeper impacts of the free sugars, monosaccharides, and disaccharides on human cells, particularly their interactions with AT. Many studies have been performed to date, mostly in vitro and on rodents. However, the experimental conditions were different across these studies, including the way in which sugar was incorporated into the diet, the gender studied, and the type of model used, along with the periodic caloric intake.

More research is still needed in this field, using clinical trials to effectively understand the impact of chronic exposure to high levels of sugar on the metabolism, with the impact on immunomodulation being especially important.

Author Contributions: Conceptualization, P.B. and E.C.; writing—original draft preparation, P.B.; writing—review and editing, P.B. and E.C. All authors have read and agreed to the published version of the manuscript.

Funding: This work was financed by the European Regional Development Fund (ERDF), through the Centro 2020 Regional Operational Programme under the project Healthy Aging 2020—CENTRO-01-0145-FEDER-000012 and through the COMPETE 2020—Operational Programme for Competitiveness and Internationalisation and Portuguese national funds via FCT—Fundação para a Ciência e a Tecnologia, under projects POCI-01-0145-FEDER-007440, UIDB/04539/2020, UIDP/04539/2020, and LA/P/0058/2020, and Pedro Barbosa's PhD grant—SFRH/BD/143849/2019.

Institutional Review Board Statement: Not applicable.

Informed Consent Statement: Not applicable.

Data Availability Statement: The data presented in this study are available on request from the corresponding author.

Conflicts of Interest: The authors declare no conflict of interest.

References

1. Kopp, W. How Western Diet and Lifestyle Drive the Pandemic of Obesity and Civilization Diseases. *Diabetes Metab. Syndr. Obes.* **2019**, *12*, 2221–2236. [CrossRef] [PubMed]
2. Amano, T.; Watanabe, D.; Otsuka, J.; Okamoto, Y.; Takada, S.; Fujii, N.; Kenny, G.P.; Enoki, Y.; Maejima, D. Comparison of hydration efficacy of carbohydrate-electrolytes beverages consisting of isomaltulose and sucrose in healthy young adults: A randomized crossover trial. *Physiol. Behav.* **2022**, *249*, 113770. [CrossRef] [PubMed]
3. Arias-Chávez, D.J.; Mailloux-Salinas, P.; Altamirano, J.; Huang, F.; Gómez-Viquez, N.L.; Bravo, G. Consumption of combined fructose and sucrose diet exacerbates oxidative stress, hypertrophy and CaMKIIδ oxidation in hearts from rats with metabolic syndrome. *Mol. Cell. Biochem.* **2022**, *477*, 1309–1320. [CrossRef] [PubMed]
4. Butterworth, P.J.; Bajka, B.H.; Edwards, C.H.; Warren, F.J.; Ellis, P.R. Enzyme kinetic approach for mechanistic insight and predictions of in vivo starch digestibility and the glycaemic index of foods. *Trends Food Sci. Technol.* **2022**, *120*, 254–264. [CrossRef]
5. Omar, N.A.M.; Frank, J.; Kruger, J.; Bello, F.D.; Medana, C.; Collino, M.; Zamaratskaia, G.; Michaelsson, K.; Wolk, A.; Landberg, R. Effects of High Intakes of Fructose and Galactose, with or without Added Fructooligosaccharides, on Metabolic Factors, Inflammation, and Gut Integrity in a Rat Model. *Mol. Nutr. Food Res.* **2021**, *65*, e2001133. [CrossRef] [PubMed]
6. Drake, I.; Sonestedt, E.; Ericson, U.; Wallström, P.; Orho-Melander, M. A Western dietary pattern is prospectively associated with cardio metabolic traits and incidence of the metabolic syndrome. *Br. J. Nutr.* **2018**, *119*, 1168–1176. [CrossRef]
7. Vasbinder, A.; Anderson, E.; Shadid, H.; Berlin, H.; Pan, M.; Azam, T.U.; Khaleel, I.; Padalia, K.; Meloche, C.; O'Hayer, P.; et al. Inflammation, Hyperglycemia, and Adverse Outcomes in Individuals With Diabetes Mellitus Hospitalized for COVID-19. *Diabetes Care* **2022**, *45*, 692–700. [CrossRef]
8. Pepin, A.; Stanhope, K.L.; Imbeault, P. Are Fruit Juices Healthier Than Sugar-Sweetened Beverages? A Review. *Nutrients* **2019**, *11*, 1006. [CrossRef]
9. Febbraio, M.A.; Karin, M. "Sweet death": Fructose as a metabolic toxin that targets the gut-liver axis. *Cell Metab.* **2021**, *33*, 2316–2328. [CrossRef]
10. McCain, H.; Kaliappan, S.; Drake, M. Invited review: Sugar reduction in dairy products. *J. Dairy Sci.* **2018**, *101*, 8619–8640. [CrossRef]
11. Patkar, O.L.; Mohamed, A.Z.; Narayanan, A.; Mardon, K.; Cowin, G.; Bhalla, R.; Stimson, D.H.R.; Kassiou, M.; Beecher, K.; Belmer, A.; et al. A binge high sucrose diet provokes systemic and cerebral inflammation in rats without inducing obesity. *Sci. Rep.* **2021**, *11*, 11252. [CrossRef] [PubMed]
12. Malik, V.S.; Popkin, B.M.; Bray, G.A.; Després, J.P.; Hu, F.B. Sugar-sweetened beverages, obesity, type 2 diabetes mellitus, and cardiovascular disease risk. *Circulation* **2010**, *121*, 1356–1364. [CrossRef] [PubMed]
13. Shendurse, A.M.; Khedkar, C.D. Lactose. *Encycl. Food Health* **2016**, 509–516. [CrossRef]
14. Meyers, A.M.; Mourra, D.; Beeler, J.A. High fructose corn syrup induces metabolic dysregulation and altered dopamine signaling in the absence of obesity. *PLoS ONE* **2017**, *12*, e0190206. [CrossRef]
15. Taskinen, M.-R.; Packard, C.J.; Borén, J. Dietary Fructose and the Metabolic Syndrome. *Nutrients* **2019**, *11*, 1987. [CrossRef]
16. Krycer, J.R.; Quek, L.-E.; Francis, D.; Zadoorian, A.; Weiss, F.C.; Cooke, K.C.; Nelson, M.E.; Diaz-Vegas, A.; Humphrey, S.J.; Scalzo, R.; et al. Insulin signaling requires glucose to promote lipid anabolism in adipocytes. *J. Biol. Chem.* **2020**, *295*, 13250–13266. [CrossRef]

17. Blanco, A.; Blanco, G. Carbohydrates. In *Medical Biochemistry*; Elsevier: Amsterdam, Netherlands, 2022; pp. 77–103. [CrossRef]
18. Olofsson, C.; Eriksson, M.; Helin, A.-C.B.; Anderstam, B.; Orsini, N.; Stenvinkel, P.; Ekberg, N.R. Effects of Acute Fructose Loading on Markers of Inflammation—A Pilot Study. *Nutrients* **2021**, *13*, 3110. [CrossRef]
19. Hannou, S.A.; Haslam, D.E.; McKeown, N.M.; Herman, M.A. Fructose metabolism and metabolic disease. *J. Clin. Investig.* **2018** *128*, 545–555. [CrossRef]
20. Legeza, B.; Marcolongo, P.; Gamberucci, A.; Varga, V.; Bánhegyi, G.; Benedetti, A.; Odermatt, A. Fructose, Glucocorticoids and Adipose Tissue: Implications for the Metabolic Syndrome. *Nutrients* **2017**, *9*, 426. [CrossRef]
21. Stanhope, K.L.; Schwarz, J.M.; Keim, N.L.; Griffen, S.C.; Bremer, A.A.; Graham, J.L.; Hatcher, B.; Cox, C.L.; Dyachenko, A.; Zhang, W.; et al. Consuming fructose-sweetened, not glucose-sweetened, beverages increases visceral adiposity and lipids and decreases insulin sensitivity in overweight/obese humans. *J. Clin. Investig.* **2009**, *119*, 1322–1334. [CrossRef]
22. Varma, V.; Boros, L.G.; Nolen, G.T.; Chang, C.-W.; Wabitsch, M.; Beger, R.D.; Kaput, J. Metabolic fate of fructose in human adipocytes: A targeted 13C tracer fate association study. *Metabolomics* **2015**, *11*, 529–544. [CrossRef] [PubMed]
23. Varma, V.; Boros, L.G.; Nolen, G.T.; Chang, C.-W.; Wabitsch, M.; Beger, R.D.; Kaput, J. Fructose Alters Intermediary Metabolism of Glucose in Human Adipocytes and Diverts Glucose to Serine Oxidation in the One–Carbon Cycle Energy Producing Pathway. *Metabolites* **2015**, *5*, 364–385. [CrossRef] [PubMed]
24. Tedeschi, P.M.; Markert, E.K.; Gounder, M.; Lin, H.; Dvorzhinski, D.; Dolfi, S.C.; Chan, L.L.Y.; Qiu, J.; DiPaola, R.S.; Hirshfield, K.M.; et al. Contribution of serine, folate and glycine metabolism to the ATP, NADPH and purine requirements of cancer cells *Cell Death Dis.* **2013**, *4*, e877. [CrossRef] [PubMed]
25. Pektas, M.B.; Koca, H.B.; Sadi, G.; Akar, F. Dietary Fructose Activates Insulin Signaling and Inflammation in Adipose Tissue: Modulatory Role of Resveratrol. *BioMed Res. Int.* **2016**, *2016*, 8014252. [CrossRef]
26. Rodrigues, D.F.; Henriques, M.C.D.C.; Oliveira, M.C.; Menezes-Garcia, Z.; Marques, P.E.; Souza, D.D.G.; Menezes, G.B.; Teixeira, M.M.; Ferreira, A.V.M. Acute intake of a high-fructose diet alters the balance of adipokine concentrations and induces neutrophil influx in the liver. *J. Nutr. Biochem.* **2014**, *25*, 388–394. [CrossRef]
27. Zhang, D.-M.; Jiao, R.-Q.; Kong, L.-D. High Dietary Fructose: Direct or Indirect Dangerous Factors Disturbing Tissue and Organ Functions. *Nutrients* **2017**, *9*, 335. [CrossRef]
28. DiNicolantonio, J.J.; Mehta, V.; Onkaramurthy, N.; O'Keefe, J.H. Fructose-induced inflammation and increased cortisol: A new mechanism for how sugar induces visceral adiposity. *Prog. Cardiovasc. Dis.* **2018**, *61*, 3–9. [CrossRef]
29. Marek, G.; Pannu, V.; Shanmugham, P.; Pancione, B.; Mascia, D.; Crosson, S.; Ishimoto, T.; Sautin, Y.Y. Adiponectin Resistance and Proinflammatory Changes in the Visceral Adipose Tissue Induced by Fructose Consumption via Ketohexokinase-Dependent Pathway. *Diabetes* **2015**, *64*, 508–518. [CrossRef]
30. Kovačević, S.; Brkljačić, J.; Milutinović, D.V.; Gligorovska, L.; Bursać, B.; Elaković, I.; Djordjevic, A. Fructose Induces Visceral Adipose Tissue Inflammation and Insulin Resistance Even Without Development of Obesity in Adult Female but Not in Male Rats. *Front. Nutr.* **2021**, *8*, 749328. [CrossRef]
31. Wang, Y.; Qi, W.; Song, G.; Pang, S.; Peng, Z.; Li, Y.; Wang, P. High-Fructose Diet Increases Inflammatory Cytokines and Alters Gut Microbiota Composition in Rats. *Mediat. Inflamm.* **2020**, *2020*, 6672636. [CrossRef]
32. Alkhouri, N.; Dixon, L.J.; Feldstein, A.E. Lipotoxicity in nonalcoholic fatty liver disease: Not all lipids are created equal. *Expert Rev. Gastroenterol. Hepatol.* **2009**, *3*, 445–451. [CrossRef]
33. Della Corte, K.W.; Perrar, I.; Penczynski, K.J.; Schwingshackl, L.; Herder, C.; Buyken, A.E. Effect of dietary sugar intake on biomarkers of subclinical inflammation: A systematic review and meta-analysis of intervention studies. *Nutrients* **2018**, *10*, 606. [CrossRef] [PubMed]
34. Jaiswal, N.; Agrawal, S.; Agrawal, A. High fructose-induced metabolic changes enhance inflammation in human dendritic cells. *Clin. Exp. Immunol.* **2019**, *197*, 237–249. [CrossRef] [PubMed]
35. Pimentel, G.; Burton, K.J.; Rosikiewicz, M.; Freiburghaus, C.; von Ah, U.; Münger, L.H.; Pralong, F.P.; Vionnet, N.; Greub, G.; Badertscher, R.; et al. Blood lactose after dairy product intake in healthy men. *Br. J. Nutr.* **2017**, *118*, 1070–1077. [CrossRef] [PubMed]
36. Conte, F.; van Buuringen, N.; Voermans, N.C.; Lefeber, D.J. Galactose in human metabolism, glycosylation and congenital metabolic diseases: Time for a closer look. *Biochim. et Biophys. Acta (BBA) Gen. Subj.* **2021**, *1865*, 129898. [CrossRef] [PubMed]
37. Krycer, J.R.; Elkington, S.D.; Diaz-Vegas, A.; Cooke, K.C.; Burchfield, J.G.; Fisher-Wellman, K.H.; Cooney, G.J.; Fazakerley, D.J.; James, D.E. Mitochondrial oxidants, but not respiration, are sensitive to glucose in adipocytes. *J. Biol. Chem.* **2020**, *295*, 99–110. [CrossRef] [PubMed]
38. Krishna, M.S.; Revathy, V.M.; Jaleel, A. Adipocytes utilize sucrose as an energy source—Effect of different carbohydrates on adipocyte differentiation. *J. Cell. Physiol.* **2020**, *235*, 891–899. [CrossRef] [PubMed]
39. Remigante, A.; Morabito, R.; Spinelli, S.; Trichilo, V.; Loddo, S.; Sarikas, A.; Dossena, S.; Marino, A. D-Galactose Decreases Anion Exchange Capability through Band 3 Protein in Human Erythrocytes. *Antioxidants* **2020**, *9*, 689. [CrossRef]
40. Hajam, Y.A.; Rani, R.; Ganie, S.Y.; Sheikh, T.A.; Javaid, D.; Qadri, S.S.; Pramodh, S.; Alsulimani, A.; Alkhanani, M.F.; Harakeh, S.; et al. Oxidative Stress in Human Pathology and Aging: Molecular Mechanisms and Perspectives. *Cells* **2022**, *11*, 552. [CrossRef]
41. Umbayev, B.; Askarova, S.; Almabayeva, A.; Saliev, T.; Masoud, A.-R.; Bulanin, D. Galactose-Induced Skin Aging: The Role of Oxidative Stress. *Oxidative Med. Cell. Longev.* **2020**, *2020*, 7145656. [CrossRef]

42. Sasaoka, N.; Imamura, H.; Kakizuka, A. A Trace Amount of Galactose, a Major Component of Milk Sugar, Allows Maturation of Glycoproteins during Sugar Starvation. *Iscience* **2018**, *10*, 211–221. [CrossRef]
43. Bouwman, L.M.S.; Fernández-Calleja, J.M.S.; van der Stelt, I.; Oosting, A.; Keijer, J.; van Schothorst, E.M. Replacing Part of Glucose with Galactose in the Postweaning Diet Protects Female But Not Male Mice from High-Fat Diet–Induced Adiposity in Later Life. *J. Nutr.* **2019**, *149*, 1140–1148. [CrossRef] [PubMed]
44. Kanuri, G.; Spruss, A.; Wagnerberger, S.; Bischoff, S.C.; Bergheim, I. Role of tumor necrosis factor α (TNFα) in the onset of fructose-induced nonalcoholic fatty liver disease in mice. *J. Nutr. Biochem.* **2011**, *22*, 527–534. [CrossRef] [PubMed]
45. Pan, L.-L.; Deng, Y.-Y.; Wang, R.; Wu, C.; Li, J.; Niu, W.; Yang, Q.; Bhatia, M.; Gudmundsson, G.H.; Agerberth, B.; et al. Lactose Induces Phenotypic and Functional Changes of Neutrophils and Macrophages to Alleviate Acute Pancreatitis in Mice. *Front. Immunol.* **2018**, *9*, 751. [CrossRef] [PubMed]
46. Paasela, M.; Kolho, K.-L.; Vaarala, O.; Honkanen, J. Lactose inhibits regulatory T-cell-mediated suppression of effector T-cell interferon-γ and IL-17 production. *Br. J. Nutr.* **2014**, *112*, 1819–1825. [CrossRef]
47. Jones, N.; Blagih, J.; Zani, F.; Rees, A.; Hill, D.G.; Jenkins, B.J.; Bull, C.J.; Moreira, D.; Bantan, A.I.M.; Cronin, J.G.; et al. Fructose reprogrammes glutamine-dependent oxidative metabolism to support LPS-induced inflammation. *Nat. Commun.* **2021**, *12*, 1209. [CrossRef]
48. Braun, C.; Weichhart, T. mTOR-dependent immunometabolism as Achilles' heel of anticancer therapy. *Eur. J. Immunol.* **2021**, *51*, 3161–3175. [CrossRef]
49. Hortová-Kohoutková, M.; Lázničková, P.; Frič, J. How immune-cell fate and function are determined by metabolic pathway choice: The bioenergetics underlying the immune response. *BioEssays* **2021**, *43*, e2000067. [CrossRef]
50. Menk, A.V.; Scharping, N.E.; Moreci, R.S.; Zeng, X.; Guy, C.; Salvatore, S.; Bae, H.; Xie, J.; Young, H.A.; Wendell, S.G.; et al. Early TCR Signaling Induces Rapid Aerobic Glycolysis Enabling Distinct Acute T Cell Effector Functions. *Cell Rep.* **2018**, *22*, 1509–1521. [CrossRef]
51. Lee, M.K.S.; Al-Sharea, A.; Shihata, W.A.; Veiga, C.B.; Cooney, O.D.; Fleetwood, A.J.; Flynn, M.C.; Claeson, E.; Palmer, C.S.; Lancaster, G.I.; et al. Glycolysis Is Required for LPS-Induced Activation and Adhesion of Human CD14+CD16− Monocytes. *Front. Immunol.* **2019**, *10*, 2054. [CrossRef]
52. Pan, J.H.; Kim, H.-S.; Beane, K.E.; Montalbano, A.M.; Lee, J.H.; Kim, Y.J.; Kim, J.H.; Kong, B.C.; Kim, S.; Park, J.-W.; et al. IDH2 Deficiency Aggravates Fructose-Induced NAFLD by Modulating Hepatic Fatty Acid Metabolism and Activating Inflammatory Signaling in Female Mice. *Nutrients* **2018**, *10*, 679. [CrossRef] [PubMed]
53. He, J.; Jiao, X.; Sun, X.; Huang, Y.; Xu, P.; Xue, Y.; Fu, T.; Liu, J.; Li, Z. Short-Term High Fructose Intake Impairs Diurnal Oscillations in the Murine Cornea. *Investig. Opthalmology Vis. Sci.* **2021**, *62*, 22. [CrossRef] [PubMed]
54. Gambaro, S.E.; Zubiría, M.G.; Portales, A.E.; Rey, M.A.; Rumbo, M.; Giovambattista, A. M1 macrophage subtypes activation and adipocyte dysfunction worsen during prolonged consumption of a fructose-rich diet. *J. Nutr. Biochem.* **2018**, *61*, 173–182. [CrossRef] [PubMed]
55. Leibowitz, A.; Rehman, A.; Paradis, P.; Schiffrin, E.L. Role of T Regulatory Lymphocytes in the Pathogenesis of High-Fructose Diet–Induced Metabolic Syndrome. *Hypertension* **2013**, *61*, 1316–1321. [CrossRef] [PubMed]
56. Lee, E.; Kim, N.; Kang, J.; Yoon, S.; Lee, H.-A.; Jung, H.; Kim, S.-H.; Kim, I. Activated pathogenic Th17 lymphocytes induce hypertension following high-fructose intake in Dahl salt-sensitive (SS) but not Dahl salt-resistant (SR) rats. *Dis. Model. Mech.* **2020**, *13*, dmm044107. [CrossRef] [PubMed]
57. Sasoh, T.; Kugo, H.; Kondo, Y.; Miyamoto, K.; Minami, M.; Higashihara, M.; Kawamoto, H.; Takeshita, F.; Moriyama, T.; Zaima, N. Different effects of high-fat and high-sucrose diets on the physiology of perivascular adipose tissues of the thoracic and abdominal aorta. *Adipocyte* **2021**, *10*, 412–423. [CrossRef]
58. Lawless, S.J.; Kedia-Mehta, N.; Walls, J.F.; McGarrigle, R.; Convery, O.; Sinclair, L.V.; Navarro, M.N.; Murray, J.; Finlay, D.K. Glucose represses dendritic cell-induced T cell responses. *Nat. Commun.* **2017**, *8*, 15620. [CrossRef]
59. Zhu, J.; Yang, W.; Zhou, X.; Zöphel, D.; Soriano-Baguet, L.; Dolgener, D.; Carlein, C.; Hof, C.; Zhao, R.; Ye, S.; et al. High Glucose Enhances Cytotoxic T Lymphocyte-Mediated Cytotoxicity. *Front. Immunol.* **2021**, *12*, 689337. [CrossRef]
60. Castro, M.C.; Villagarcía, H.; Nazar, A.; Arbeláez, L.G.; Massa, M.L.; Del Zotto, H.; Ríos, J.L.; Schinella, G.; Francini, F. Cacao extract enriched in polyphenols prevents endocrine-metabolic disturbances in a rat model of prediabetes triggered by a sucrose rich diet. *J. Ethnopharmacol.* **2020**, *247*, 112263. [CrossRef]
61. Millet, P.; Vachharajani, V.; McPhail, L.; Yoza, B.; McCall, C.E. GAPDH Binding to TNF-α mRNA Contributes to Posttranscriptional Repression in Monocytes: A Novel Mechanism of Communication between Inflammation and Metabolism. *J. Immunol.* **2016**, *196*, 2541–2551. [CrossRef]
62. Hasegawa, H.; Matsumoto, T. Mechanisms of Tolerance Induction by Dendritic Cells In Vivo. *Front. Immunol.* **2018**, *9*, 350. [CrossRef] [PubMed]
63. Bhattacharjee, J.; Kumar, J.M.; Arindkar, S.; Das, B.; Pramod, U.; Juyal, R.C.; Majumdar, S.S.; Nagarajan, P. Role of immunodeficient animal models in the development of fructose induced NAFLD. *J. Nutr. Biochem.* **2014**, *25*, 219–226. [CrossRef] [PubMed]
64. Nishimura, S.; Manabe, I.; Nagasaki, M.; Eto, K.; Yamashita, H.; Ohsugi, M.; Otsu, M.; Hara, K.; Ueki, K.; Sugiura, S.; et al. CD8+ effector T cells contribute to macrophage recruitment and adipose tissue inflammation in obesity. *Nat. Med.* **2009**, *15*, 914–920. [CrossRef] [PubMed]

65. Lynch, L.A.; O'Connell, J.M.; Kwasnik, A.K.; Cawood, T.J.; O'Farrelly, C.; O'Shea, D. Are Natural Killer Cells Protecting the Metabolically Healthy Obese Patient? *Obesity* **2009**, *17*, 601–605. [CrossRef] [PubMed]
66. Zhang, D.; Jin, W.; Wu, R.; Li, J.; Park, S.-A.; Tu, E.; Zanvit, P.; Xu, J.; Liu, O.; Cain, A.; et al. High Glucose Intake Exacerbates Autoimmunity through Reactive-Oxygen-Species-Mediated TGF-β Cytokine Activation. *Immunity* **2019**, *51*, 671–681.e5. [CrossRef] [PubMed]
67. Zeng, H.; Chi, H. The interplay between regulatory T cells and metabolism in immune regulation. *Oncoimmunology* **2013**, *2*, e26586. [CrossRef] [PubMed]

diabetology

MDPI

Review

The Bitter Side of Sugar Consumption: A Mitochondrial Perspective on Diabetes Development

Mariana S. Diniz [1,2], Carolina Tocantins [1,2], Luís F. Grilo [1,2] and Susana P. Pereira [1,3,*]

1 CNC—Center for Neuroscience and Cell Biology, CIBB—Centre for Innovative Biomedicine and Biotechnology, University of Coimbra, 3004-531 Coimbra, Portugal
2 PhD Programme in Experimental Biology and Biomedicine (PDBEB), Institute for Interdisciplinary Research (IIIUC), University of Coimbra, 3004-531 Coimbra, Portugal
3 Laboratory of Metabolism and Exercise (LaMetEx), Research Centre in Physical Activity, Health and Leisure (CIAFEL), Laboratory for Integrative and Translational Research in Population Health (ITR), Faculty of Sports, University of Porto, 4099-002 Porto, Portugal
* Correspondence: pereirasusan@gmail.com; Tel.: +351-231-249-170

Abstract: Type 2 diabetes (T2D) has increased worldwide at an alarming rate. Metabolic syndrome (MetS) is a major risk factor for T2D development. One of the main reasons for the abrupt rise in MetS incidence, besides a sedentary lifestyle, is the westernized diet consumption, with high content of industrialized foods, rich in added dietary sugars (DS), mainly sucrose and fructose. It has been suggested that a higher intake of DS could impair metabolic function, inducing MetS, and predisposing to T2D. However, it remains poorly explored how excessive DS intake modulates mitochondrial function, a key player in metabolism. This review explores the relationship between increased consumption of DS and mitochondrial dysfunction associated with T2D development, pointing to a contribution of the diet-induced accumulation of advanced glycation end-products (AGEs), with brief insights on the impact of maternal high-sugar diet and AGEs consumption during gestation on offspring increased risk of developing T2D later in life, contributing to perpetuate T2D propagation.

Keywords: industrialized food; dietary sugars; metabolic dysfunction; maternal high-sugar diet; disease programming

Citation: Diniz, M.S.; Tocantins, C.; Grilo, L.F.; Pereira, S.P. The Bitter Side of Sugar Consumption: A Mitochondrial Perspective on Diabetes Development. *Diabetology* **2022**, 3, 583–595. https://doi.org/10.3390/diabetology3040044

Academic Editor: Peter Clifton

Received: 30 September 2022
Accepted: 1 November 2022
Published: 7 November 2022

Publisher's Note: MDPI stays neutral with regard to jurisdictional claims in published maps and institutional affiliations.

1. Introduction

1.1. Metabolic Syndrome Development: The Case of Type 2 Diabetes

The Metabolic Syndrome (MetS) affects around 35% of the adult population in the United States, about 40% in Europe, between 20.7% and 42.7% in the Middle East, and up to 58.1% in >60 age Chinese population [1]. Each region adopts different diagnostic criteria for MetS without general consensus in the medical community [2,3].

The MetS is characterized by a set of metabolic disorders, including dyslipidemia, hypertension, insulin resistance (IR), visceral adipose tissue (VAT) dysfunction, and VAT-related endocrine mediation [3]. Systemic pathophysiological responses are then activated, such as endothelial dysfunction, chronic inflammation, oxidative stress and atherothrombosis [3,4].

Due to the MetS-associated pathophysiology, MetS is one of the major risk factors for type 2 diabetes (T2D) and cardiovascular disease (CVD) development [1,4]. MetS is associated with a 1.36 increased risk of cardiovascular death, 1.46-fold risk of myocardial infarction, 1.43-fold risk of stroke, and 2.92-fold of T2D [5,6].

Distinct components of the MetS have a different impact in T2D development-risk [7]. Among the MetS predisposing factors (e.g., genetic, environmental), diet and sedentary behaviors have been pointed out as the most relevant [3]. The critical role of diet in MetS extends not only to the unbalanced energy intake vs. expenditure but also to the composition of the diets, such as the western diet (WD) which is rich in saturated and unsaturated fats, simple carbohydrates, and poor in fibers, including red meat, processed foods rich in ultra-processed carbohydrates and fats, and re-packaged foods [8].

1.2. The Bitter Risks of Increased Dietary Sugars Consumption

Dietary sugars (DS) correspond to the sugar content of foods that comprehend the sugars naturally present in the food and the sugars added to foods during processing or preparation. Sugars can be labeled as "free sugars" and "intrinsic sugars". Intrinsic sugars are encapsulated by a cell wall, such as the ones present in brown rice, whole fruit, vegetables, etc. [9]. These tend to be digested at a lower rate and take longer to enter the bloodstream in comparison with "free sugars" [9]. On the contrary, "free sugars" have been refined to some extent, and are not present inside the cells of the food consumed, comprising all the monosaccharides (i.e., glucose, fructose, and galactose) and disaccharides (i.e., sucrose, lactose, and maltose) added to foods by the manufacturer, cook, or consumer, plus sugars present in honey, syrups, and unsweetened fruit juices [9]. Altogether, all naturally-occurring sugars along with the added sugars compose the "total sugars" [10,11].

Sugars can also be referred to as carbohydrates. Carbohydrates encompass the sugars, starches, and dietary fibers that naturally exist in plant-based foods and dairy products, being one of the main energy sources for the human body. During digestion, the carbohydrates are broken down into simple sugars, raising monosaccharides' blood concentrations. The carbohydrate's glycemic index (GI) represents the respective increase in blood glucose after the intake of carbohydrates and appears to be critical to define the most concerning classes of sugars. While low GI foods are rich in dietary fibers and induce lower concentrations of fasting triglycerides and LDL-cholesterol, a high intake of elevated GI foods causes IR and contributes to T2D [3].

General consumption of sugars has been rising worldwide over the last decades [12,13]. A primary concern is sugar-sweetened beverages, for which sweeteners are commonly sucrose (composed of glucose and fructose) and corn syrup (rich in fructose) [13]. Fructose overconsumption is a significant driver of MetS development due to its unique metabolization, almost exclusively in the enterocytes and liver, capable of bypassing the hormonal and metabolic regulatory control [13]. Sugar-sweetened beverages and other high energy-dense drinks have a moderate-to-high GI while decreasing satiety and impairing compensatory energy intake [14]. The consumption of these beverages has been associated with T2D development [14].

Nevertheless, the causal relationship between sugar consumption and T2D development has not been scientifically demonstrated. Most of the studies show that the effect of sugars on long-term T2D development is not driven by a direct impact of sugars in the disease pathophysiology, but rather by the promotion of T2D risk factors, such as extra calorie intake, obesity, and MetS that later can lead to IR and T2D phenotype [10]. One possible driver behind this relationship is systemic inflammation which mediators increase due to free-fructose overconsumption [15]. This mechanism, however, seems to be shared by other dietary sugars [16].

Most of the studies point out that, from a sugar-induced disease perspective, the sugar source is not the most important aspect, including sweetened beverages or fruit juices [17–19]. Despite more studies being required, mostly related to cellular responses rather than blood parameters and metabolites' landscape, the general literature states that sugar consumption has a modest impact on immediate glycemic control [17,20].

It is important to note that high sugar-containing foods are one of the main sources of energy in infants, children, and adolescents [21], either as a snack or after a regular meal, which contributes to a critically high GI and increased calorie intake, promoting T2D development at early life stages. The hormonal, metabolic, and lifestyle alterations characteristic of adolescence represent a critical period for metabolic disease development, becoming a priority to focus studies on the impact of DS consumption at early ages.

2. The Impact of Dietary Sugars on Mitochondrial Function and Promotion of Type 2 Diabetes

The cellular metabolism of sugars, fats, and amino acids results in chemical energy production in the form of adenosine triphosphate (ATP), mainly by mitochondria [22]. Mitochondria are multifaceted organelles and cellular energy metabolism highly relies on mitochondrial function [22]. Impaired mitochondrial function has been associated with IR mechanisms, ultimately leading to T2D development [23]. In T2D, mitochondrial dysfunction is characterized by decreased electron transport chain (ETC) complexes expression and activity, slower respiration, lower organelle density, decreased ATP maximum synthesis rate, increased reactive oxygen species (ROS) production, and impaired mitochondrial dynamics, with an increased rate of fission events [23]. This has been vastly reported across several organs such as the skeletal muscle, adipose tissue, liver, and heart [23]. Nevertheless, the impact of DS, namely fructose, on mitochondrial function has been poorly explored. The current section will disclose the current knowledge on the impact of DS in mitochondria across several tissues, especially in the liver and the heart, and how mitochondrial dysfunction induced by excessive ingestion of DS, especially fructose, could prompt T2D development (Figures 1 and 2).

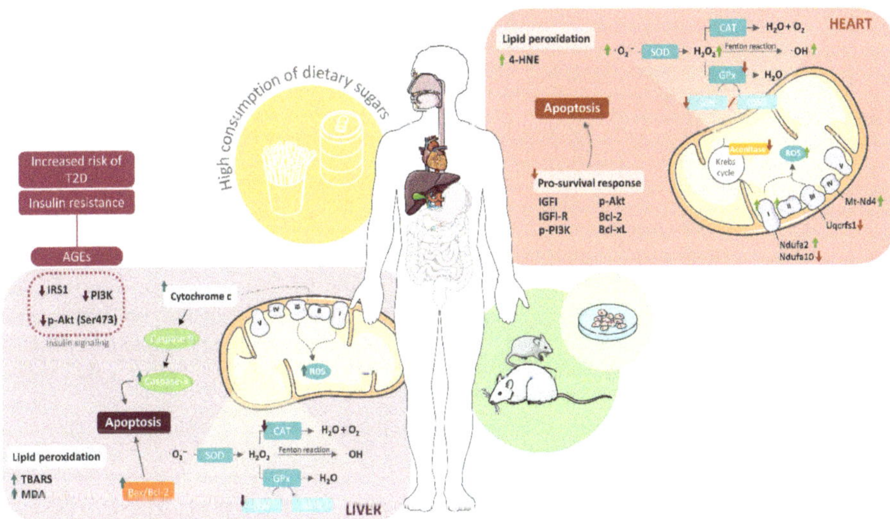

Figure 1. Metabolic alterations induced by high consumption of dietary sugars in the liver and the heart, contributing to mitochondrial dysfunction and the development of risk factors associated with type 2 diabetes (T2D) development. Increased consumption of dietary sugars, especially fructose, leads to impaired mitochondrial respiratory chain function, resulting in altered activity and protein levels of the mitochondrial oxidative phosphorylation system, namely in the subunits of the electron transport chain (I–IV) in the heart. Such alterations contribute to increased reactive oxygen species (ROS) production and inefficient response of the antioxidant defenses. Oxidative stress can induce an apoptotic response by dysregulation of pro-survival and pro-apoptotic proteins. Lipid peroxidation, which contributes to cell damage, is also a result of augmented oxidative stress. Increased levels of advanced glycation end-products (AGEs) interfere with the expression of proteins involved in the insulin signaling pathway, which may promote insulin resistance, a prime risk factor for T2D. IRS1–insulin receptor substrate 1, PI3K-phosphoinositide 3-kinase, Akt–protein kinase B, TBARS-thiobarbituric acid reactive substances, MDA–malondialdehyde, SOD–superoxide dismutase, CAT–catalase, GPx–glutathione peroxidase, 4-HNE-4-Hydroxynonenal, IGFI-insulin-like growth factor 1, IGFI-R–IGFI receptor, GSH–reduced glutathione, GSSG–glutathione disulfide, NDUFA2/10-NADH dehydrogenase [ubiquinone] 1 alpha subcomplex subunits 2 and 10, UQCRFS1-ubiquinol-cytochrome *c* reductase iron-sulfur subunit 1, MT-ND4-mitochondrially encoded NADH: ubiquinone oxidoreductase core subunit 4.

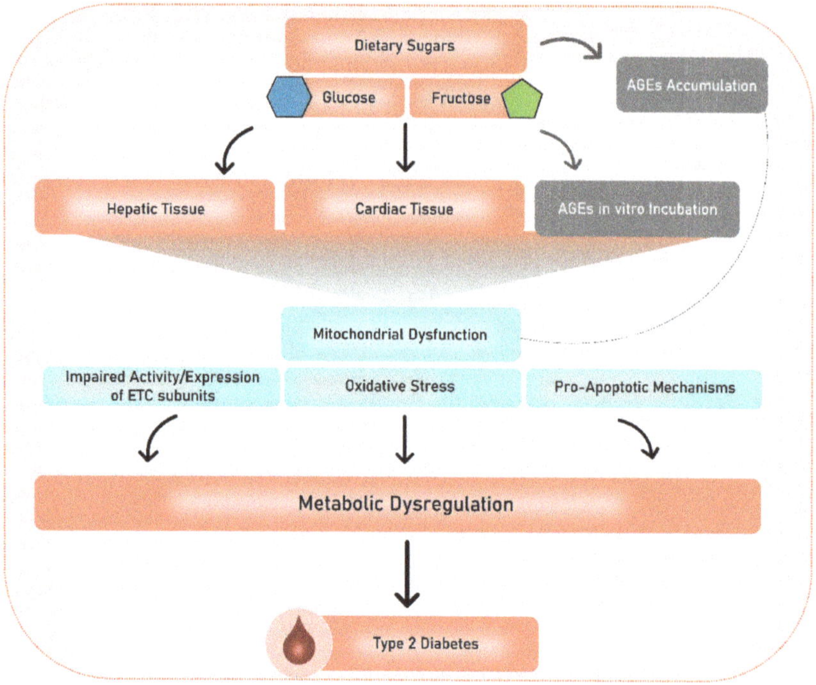

Figure 2. Increased intake of dietary sugars (mainly glucose and fructose) leads to mitochondrial dysfunction. Mitochondrial dysfunction across hepatic and cardiac tissue triggers metabolic dysregulation, including insulin resistance, which ultimately induces the development of type 2 diabetes. In parallel, it is hypothesized that advanced glycation end-products (AGEs) accumulation induced by higher consumption of dietary sugars could lead to mitochondrial dysfunction, through AGEs receptors (RAGEs) activation. Evidence shows that in vitro incubation of different cell lines either with AGEs precursors or AGEs, results in mitochondrial dysfunction, which could act as a starting point to induced metabolic dysregulation and induces type 2 diabetes development.

2.1. High-Fructose Intake and Mitochondrial Function Modulation

The first step of fructose metabolism requires ATP utilization by the enzyme fructokinase. An exacerbated intake of fructose leads to increasing demand for ATP utilization by the organs [24]. This could be the origin of increased electron flow through the mitochondrial ETC [25,26]. As insulin-sensitive organs, the liver and the heart are of particular interest to study alterations predisposing to T2D. Indeed, in Sprague-Dawley rats, the intake of free high fructose (HFr) for 6 weeks, impairs the activity of mitochondrial ETC, increasing complex-I activity in the heart [27], and 20-week-free HFr treatment decreased complex-II activity in isolated cardiac mitochondria, with decreased mitochondrial oxygen consumption rates and ATP-linked oxygen consumption (state 3–stimulated by the addition of fuel substrates, supports coupled energy conversion) [28,29]. Along with this, proteomic analysis of Wistar rats cardiac tissue after a 24-week HFr-diet identified alterations in the subunits of the ETC, with increased protein content of complex-I, and IV (NDUFA2, Mt-ND4) and decreased complex-I, and III (NDUFA10, UQCRFS1) subunits [29]. In the hepatic tissue, free-HFr treatment for 6 weeks also induced ETC impairment with hepatic mitochondria from free HFr-fed Wistar rats presenting decreased ATP-linked oxygen consumption [30]. HFr diet induced-dysfunctional mitochondrial ETC, with impaired respiration, could induce increased electron escaping through the ETC complexes-I and III, prompting altered mitochondrial membrane potential along with increased electron reactivity with oxygen, leading to an overproduction of ROS, which ultimately could produce biomolecules' oxidative damage. Indeed, evidence of redox imbalance has been reported in the hepatic and cardiac tissues of HFr-fed murine animal models, independently of the duration and type of HFr treatment. In the liver and heart of dietary HFr/free-HFr fed-rats, lipid peroxidation is increased, demonstrated by increased levels of thiobarbituric acid (TBARS) [31,32], malondialdehyde (MDA) [33], and 4-Hydroxynonenal (4-HNE) [27,32]. In other respects, hepatic antioxidant defenses are diminished, as indicated by decreased superoxide dismutase (SOD) [32] and GSH-S transferase activities [33], lower protein levels of glutathione peroxidase 1 (GPx1) [27], reduced GSH/GSSG ratio [27,28], and diminished catalase activity [34]. In addition, increased production of ROS, assessed through increased superoxide and hydroxyl radicals [28], augmented hydrogen peroxide production [28], and decreased aconitase activity were verified in hepatic and cardiac tissues from HFr-fed rats [27].

Pro-apoptotic mechanisms can be activated by increased oxidative injury [35]. High fructose-induced alterations of proteins involved in cell apoptosis and survival, which are mediated by cell signaling cascades, have been mightily documented in the hearts and livers of HFr-fed murine animal models. An increased number of apoptotic cells has been reported in the cardiac tissue of HFr-fed Wistar rats [36], hepatic tissue of mice [35], and in cardiomyocytes differentiated from an H9C2 rat-myoblastic cell line [37] through the TUNEL assay or DNA strand break labeling, along with increased levels of the activated form of caspase-3 [34], Bax and increased Bax/BcL-2 ratio [33] and cytosolic cytochrome *c* amount [33]. All of these mechanisms are critically involved in the intrinsic mitochondrial apoptotic pathway [31]. Consistently, reports described HFr-induced suppression of pro-survival mechanisms–so-called due to its ability to negatively regulate pro-apoptotic mechanisms, by suppressing the activation of caspases and pro-apoptotic proteins, as confirmed by decreased activation of PI3K and Akt and/or expression levels of the pro-survival proteins, IGFI, IGFI-R, Bcl-2, and Bcl-xL in the cardiac tissues of HFr-fed Wistar rats [36]. Moreover, during the process of apoptosis, it has been reported that mitochondrial dynamics machinery disintegrates for cytochrome *c* release. Mitochondrial kinetics comprehend motility, fusion, fission, biogenesis, and mitophagy. The equilibrium between these processes allows the preservation of mitochondrial number, and morphology and impacts mitochondrial function. Mitochondrial fusion consists of the merging of two adjacent mitochondria. This process can be used, up to a certain level, to alleviate stress by combining the content of partially damaged mitochondria. Mitochondrial fusion is coordinated by proteins that bind and promote membrane fusion, including mitofusin (MFN)- 1 and 2 [38,39]. On the contrary, mitochondrial fission is the mechanism that generates mitochondrial fragmentation; it is driven by proteins that first direct the constriction of membranes and then mitochondrial splitting, including mitochondrial fission factor (MFF), a tail-anchored protein of the mitochondrial outer membrane that acts as the receptor for dynamin-related protein-1 (DRP1), a cytosolic GTPase that tends to oligomerize. The mitochondrial fission protein 1 (FIS1) has been also implicated in mitochondrial fission [38,39]. This process is essential for mitochondrial duplication, but also for the clearance of damaged mitochondria during high levels of cellular stress [38,39]. Thus, maintaining a balance between fission and fusion events is essential to sustain mitochondrial integrity and homeostasis. Several proteins involved in mitochondrial fission and fusion events have been pointed out to act as apoptosis inductors, especially DRP1, which is involved in cytochrome *c* release, FIS1, which is involved in Bax translocation, and optic atrophy 1 (OPA1), which, conversely, prevents mitochondrial fission, protecting cells from apoptosis [40]. It has been shown that primary cell lines treated with glucose, one of the main dietary sugars, exhibit increased mitochondrial fragmentation, which has been suggested to be mediated by hyperglycemia-induced modulation of fission and fusion proteins [41]. Indeed, human umbilical vein-derived endothelial cells (HUVECs) treated with high glucose levels present signs of mitochondrial fragmentation [42]. Cells from the cardiovascular system (i.e., neonatal rat ventricular myocytes, H9C2 cell line, bovine aortic endothelial cells, and mouse aortic smooth muscle cells) treated in hyperglycemic conditions present increased mitochondrial fragmentation, which is induced by an increased expression of the protein DRP1/DLP1, mediating hyperglycemia-induced cell death [41]. Moreover, proximal tubular cell lines (HK-2), present increased mitochondrial fragmentation induced by hyperglycemic conditions, which is preserved by the pharmacological modulation of proteins involved in mitochondrial dynamics (FIS1, DRP1, MFN1, and MFN2) [43]. These findings reflect a potential deleterious effect of dietary sugars on mitochondrial dynamics that, ultimately could cause cell death. Nevertheless, more studies are required to deepen this potential impairment and compare it to fructose-treated cell lines, along with the complementation of data from animal models treated with high-glucose/fructose diets.

Apoptosis mediated by mitochondria, in both the liver and heart, can lead to tissue inflammation and organ pathologies, ultimately affecting whole-body homeostasis. Altogether, the evidence discussed above demonstrates that the overconsumption of fructose, independently of treatment type and duration, can result in mitochondrial dysfunction, impairing cardiac and hepatic mitochondrial respiration, generating oxidative stress, dysregulating mitochondrial dynamics, and trigger programmed cell death. Nevertheless, the reason behind DS mitochondrial function impairment has not yet been fully disclosed However, recently, it has been described that mitochondrial dysfunction could be, in part, induced by an accumulation of dietary advanced glycation end-products (AGEs), due to their elevated presence in processed foods [44,45].

2.2. Advanced Glycation End-Products Accumulation Induce Mitochondrial Dysfunction: A Potential Mechanism in Type 2 Diabetes

Advanced glycation end-products have been pointed out as potential biomarkers of a diabetic condition, inducing IR and, possibly, mitochondrial dysfunction [46]. AGEs are the result of the "Maillard reaction" [47], which is described as a non-enzymatic spontaneous reaction between reducing sugars with lipids, nucleic acids, and free amino acid groups from proteins [47]. In addition, AGEs can also be a product of the oxidation of sugars, lipids, and amino acids [48]. However, reducing sugars are one of the main sources of AGEs [47]. Interestingly, in vitro observations have indicated that fructose is one of the most potent glycation agents [49]. Hyperglycemia could prompt AGEs accumulation, which could play a major pathologic role in contributing to the dysregulation of many cellular functions in the organism [50], predisposing to the development of T2D. Indeed, AGEs are toxic metabolic byproducts, and the effects of AGEs' whole-body accumulation have been documented in diverse mechanisms (i.e., de novo lipid synthesis, lipogenic pathway, inflammatory response) [49]. Specifically, the development of IR has been associated with systemic AGEs accumulation in mouse animal models and even in humans [51]. On the other hand, AGEs restriction prevents IR, highlighting the role of AGEs in the development of IR-related mechanisms [46]. Although the specific mechanisms by which AGEs induce IR remain unknown, dietary-AGEs impaired insulin signaling pathway has been verified in both in vitro and in vivo models [51]. Hepatocytes, adipocytes, and pancreatic beta cells treated with AGEs precursor [51], methylglyoxal (MG), which is a metabolite of the glycolytic pathway, show decreased activation of insulin receptor substrate 1 (IRS1), Akt phosphorylation in the Ser473 residue [51], and reduced activity of phosphoinositide 3-kinase (PI3K) [52]. Additionally, Sprague-Dawley rats with a 4-week administration of MG presented enhanced insulin resistance, which was evaluated through the euglycemic hyperinsulinemic glucose clamp technique in the circulating blood [53]. The overproduction of AGEs could also contribute to the activation of membrane receptors, such as RAGEs [26], inducing a cycle of mitochondrial dysfunction and oxidative damage, and promoting apoptosis [54]. Evidence suggests that RAGEs activation could stimulate complex-I, leading to increased ROS production, prompting the organism for oxidative stress [54]. In spite of this, decreased activities of complex-I and -IV were verified in the cerebral cortex of mice fed with a MG-rich diet [55] and in human retinal pigmented epithelium cell lines treated with AGE-BSA [56]. Nevertheless, the presence of oxidative stress is confirmed in most studies, describing increased production of superoxide anion, or hydrogen peroxide, and/or loss of MnSOD activity in the serum of MG-fed mice [55], beta cells [57], endothelial progenitor cells [54], and chondrogenic cells [56] treated with AGEs (N^{ε}-carboxymethyl lysine (CML), when mentioned [57]). Furthermore, AGEs treatment appeared to induce ATP depletion in MG-treated adipocytes [55], loss of mitochondrial membrane potential, and apoptosis, which is confirmed through increased Bax/BcL-2 ratio and increased release of cleaved caspase 3 in AGEs-treated chondrogenic ATDC5 cells [56]. Even though this has been mostly documented for in vitro models, data concerning in vivo and tissue-targeted studies is still lacking and demands further investigation so the relationship between AGEs accumulation, IR, and mitochondrial dysfunction can be established and ultimately, fully understand the contribution of AGEs accumulation and mechanism for inducing T2D development potentiating new preventative strategies for T2D development.

3. Type 2 Diabetes and Its Origin in the Womb: The Consequences of Maternal High-Sugar Diet in the Offspring's Metabolic Function

Maternal lifestyle habits, such as the type and quantity of food at preconception [58], gestation [59], and lactation [60], may influence critical periods of fetal/infant development, contributing to future offspring complications [58–61]. Maternal malnutrition is associated with an increased risk of obesity, T2D, and CVD in young and adult offspring [62–64]. Increased generalization of westernized diets, rich in added sugars, even during pregnancy turns vital to study the influence of maternal DS on the offspring's development and health. Although it is well-established that maternal high-processed fat diets programs the offspring to metabolic alterations [65,66], the lack of information concerning appropriate maternal ingestion of added sugars during gestation and/or lactation is evident [67].

While maternal high-DS consumption may be deleterious for the fetus, more human studies are needed to confirm it [68]. Resorting to studies with animal models examining this biological question, it was described that C57BL/6J mice offspring exposed to HFr during development presented increased: body-weight, blood pressure, glucose area under the curve (AUC), and adipose tissue [66,69]. Sprague-Dawley rat 90-day-old offspring plasma revealed leptinemia, increased IR, and oxidative stress markers (advanced oxidation products (AOPP) and uricemia) in male but not in female offspring [70]. However, 1-year-old C57BL/6J mice female offspring showed increased homeostasis model assessment of insulin resistance (HOMA-IR) score, elevated leptin levels, and decreased adiponectin [66]. Accordingly, 261-day-old Sprague-Dawley rat male offspring exposed to maternal HFr during pregnancy presented similar results [71]. Further analysis in the hepatic tissue showed increased expression of serine phosphorylated form of IRS2, suggesting reduced insulin signaling in the liver [71]. In another study, fetuses of HFr-fed Wistar rats throughout pregnancy until postnatal day-10 showed increased hepatic GLUT5, oppositely to fructokinase mRNA levels, and high triglycerides content [72]. Ten days postnatally, male offspring exhibited decreased expression of hepatic β-oxidation genes, while females showed augmented AMP-activated protein kinase (AMPK) transcript levels in the liver [72]. In fact, phosphorylated AMPKα was decreased in the livers of 22-day-old female offspring of fructose-treated Wistar rats during gestation [73]. Seven-month-old C57BL/6J pups exposed to maternal HFr consumption during pregnancy and lactation presented increased expression of lipogenesis-related proteins and triglycerides accumulation, contributing to altered morphology with increased liver size [69]. This suggests maternal free-HFr-supplemented diet significantly affects liver metabolism and function, predisposing the offspring to obesity, hypertension, and metabolic dysfunction, which are critical risk factors for T2D development. Nevertheless, research to unravel the cellular mechanisms involved is critically necessary.

Few studies explored the effect of maternal fructose consumption on offspring's cardiac tissue. Maternal HFr rodent supplementation resulted in 1-day-old offspring's increased expression of glucose metabolism- and insulin signaling-related genes in the heart and brain, which actively contribute to blood pressure regulation, possibly contributing to the programming of hypertension in adulthood [74]. This period is significant for the offspring's cardiac development since adaptation to the extrauterine life involves a substrate utilization shift from glucose towards fatty acids [75]. Maternal HFr diet during pregnancy and lactation led to mild myocardial hypertrophy in 3-month-old male Sprague-Dawley rat offspring, with collagen fibers deposition and marked oxidative stress in the cardiac tissue [76]. The induced cardiac fibrosis and oxidative damage exacerbated cardiac remodeling [76] for which mitochondria play a crucial role [77].

Another characteristic of WD is the concomitant high intake of AGEs. Serum AGEs (sAGEs) have been proposed to be maternally transferred through the placenta [78]. Nonetheless, the levels of sAGEs might reflect dietary AGEs consumption [79]. Young-adult offspring of C57BL/6 mice from mothers fed an AGEs-rich diet (with increased CML content) showed reduced insulin sensitivity and increased body weight [80]. As briefly mentioned, maternal diet during lactation may also affect perinatal development since it influences breast milk composition [81]. Offspring of MG-treated Wistar rat mothers developed increased body weight, adipose tissue, glucose intolerance, and β-cell dysfunction in adulthood, increasing their predisposition for T2D [81].

Concerning the consumption of DS, few studies assessed the effect of maternal diet on the offspring's mitochondrial function. Most focus on brain development and cognitive function. Brain mitochondria of aging Fischer F344 rat offspring exposed to maternal HFr showed decreased P/O_2 ratio [82]. Hippocampi mitochondria of weaned Sprague-Dawley rat offspring after exposure to maternal HFr during pregnancy and lactation showed reduced TFAM mRNA levels and compromised mitochondrial oxygen consumption rates [83]. Studies are lacking to fully understand the role of maternal DS on mitochondrial metabolism and its implications in fetal development and offspring programming of metabolic diseases in adulthood.

4. Mitochondrial-Targeted Therapies for T2D Management

The clinically well-established treatment of T2D with metformin presents the capacity of shifting the main energy substrate used across several tissues [23], the ability to modulate mitochondrial dynamics, especially mitochondrial fission events in endothelial cells, and prevent superoxide generation [23]. In addition, metformin has been suggested to inhibit mitochondrial complex-I activity, which is an extremely relevant feature from a therapeutic perspective [84].

Dietary supplementation has been also demonstrated to have positive effects in modulating mitochondrial function. For example, flavonoids from mulberry leaves have been suggested to improve skeletal muscle mitochondrial function in diabetic mice, through the modulation of the AMPK/peroxisome proliferator-activated receptor- γ coactivator 1 α axis (AMPK/PGC-1α) [85], highlighting a potential role in T2D management [85]. Other studies have suggested that by inhibiting fructose metabolism through ketohexokinase [86], the primary fructose metabolizing enzyme, and fructose-1,6-bisphosphatase [87], it could be possible to prevent the development of metabolic disease, including T2D. Both approaches seem to prevent hyperinsulinemia and hyperglycemia, thus highlighting novel therapeutic approaches to T2D. It is though relevant to mention that more straightforward approaches have been suggested, such as the removal of fructose from the diet [88]. Indeed, diet-switching reversed mitochondrial function and prevented oxidative stress in the hippocampus of Wistar rats [88]. More studies across other tissues are required to understand if mitochondrial function improvement is verified as well. Nonetheless, given that, in theory, this is a relatively simple strategy to be implemented it is highly relevant for T2D clinical management, making it worth the additional efforts to overcome the challenges of adherence to nutritional interventions, particularly during pregnancy. Given maternal HFr-induced deleterious effects on the offspring's metabolism across many tissues (Section 3), it is also worth mentioning that a study revealed that the administration of Coenzyme Q10 in the offspring, which is a key-mediator of mitochondrial ETC [89], improved mitochondrial biogenesis, and ATP levels, preventing maternal HFr-diet-induced adverse effects in the retinas of female offspring [89].

Mitochondrial-based therapies have a great potential to be explored in T2D prevention and treatment. The follow-up of these studies or new studies could give origin to improved strategies to counteract T2D, even before birth, thus reducing the global burden of this metabolic disease.

5. Conclusions

The overconsumption of free sugars significantly contributes to whole-body DS excess and could severely impact mitochondrial function through alterations in the subunits' expression levels and in the enzymatic activity of the ETC complexes, leading to oxidative stress, mitochondrial dynamics impairment, and activation of apoptotic mechanisms. DS-induced mitochondrial dysfunction can be a result of an accumulation of dietary AGEs, nevertheless, further studies are demanded to confirm this hypothesis and to establish a solid relationship between excessive DS consumption and T2D development. In addition, maternal high-sugar diet consumption impacts the offspring's metabolism at different time-points in the lifetime (i.e., fetal, neonatal, and postnatal stages), in a sex-dependent way, across different animal models, and along with increased levels of AGEs, could predispose the offspring for T2D development.

Author Contributions: All the authors have responsibility for the entire content of this manuscript and approve its submission. Conceptualization, M.S.D., C.T., L.F.G. and S.P.P.; investigation, M.S.D., C.T., L.F.G. and S.P.P.; resources, M.S.D., C.T., L.F.G. and S.P.P.; visualization, M.S.D. and C.T. writing—original draft, M.S.D., C.T. and L.F.G.; writing—review and editing, M.S.D., C.T., L.F.G. and S.P.P.; supervision—S.P.P.; project administration S.P.P. All authors have read and agreed to the published version of the manuscript.

Funding: This research was funded by the ERDF funds through the Operational Programme for Competitiveness–COMPETE 2020 and national funds by Foundation for Science and Technology under FCT-Post-doctoral Fellowship (SPP, SFRH/BPD/116061/2016), FCT-doctoral Fellowship (MSD, SFRH/BD/11934/2022; CT, SFRH/BD/11924/2022; LFG, SFRH/BD/5539/2020), project grant PTDC/DTP-DES/1082/2014 (POCI-01-0145-FEDER-016657), CENTRO-01-0246-FEDER-000010 (Multidisciplinary Institute of Ageing in Coimbra), strategic projects UIDB/04539/2020, UIDP/04539/2020, and LA/P/0058/2020, Fulbright Scholarship for Research (LFG), and Luso-American Development Foundation, R&D at USA Grant (LFG).

Institutional Review Board Statement: Not applicable.

Informed Consent Statement: Not applicable.

Data Availability Statement: The data presented in this study are available on request from the corresponding author.

Conflicts of Interest: The authors declare no conflict of interest.

References

1. McCracken, E.; Monaghan, M.; Sreenivasan, S. Pathophysiology of the Metabolic Syndrome. *Clin. Dermatol.* **2018**, *36*, 14–20. [CrossRef]
2. Lemieux, I.; Després, J.P. Metabolic Syndrome: Past, Present and Future. *Nutrients* **2020**, *12*, 3501. [CrossRef] [PubMed]
3. Bovolini, A.; Garcia, J.; Andrade, M.A.; Duarte, J.A. Metabolic Syndrome Pathophysiology and Predisposing Factors. *Int. J. Sports Med.* **2021**, *42*, 199–214. [CrossRef]
4. Gonzalez-Chávez, A.; Chávez-Fernández, J.A.; Elizondo-Argueta, S.; González-Tapia, A.; León-Pedroza, J.I.; Ochoa, C. Metabolic Syndrome and Cardiovascular Disease: A Health Challenge. *Arch. Med. Res.* **2018**, *49*, 516–521. [CrossRef] [PubMed]
5. Lee, Y.-B.; Kim, D.H.; Kim, S.M.; Kim, N.H.; Choi, K.M.; Baik, S.H.; Park, Y.G.; Han, K.; Yoo, H.J. Risk of Type 2 Diabetes According to the Cumulative Exposure to Metabolic Syndrome or Obesity: A Nationwide Population-based Study. *J. Diabetes Investig.* **2020**, *11*, 1583. [CrossRef]
6. Li, X.; Zhai, Y.; Zhao, J.; He, H.; Li, Y.; Liu, Y.; Feng, A.; Li, L.; Huang, T.; Xu, A.; et al. Impact of Metabolic Syndrome and It's Components on Prognosis in Patients with Cardiovascular Diseases: A Meta-Analysis. *Front. Cardiovasc. Med.* **2021**, *8*, 704145. [CrossRef]
7. Marott, S.C.W.; Nordestgaard, B.G.; Tybjærg-Hansen, A.; Benn, M. Components of the Metabolic Syndrome and Risk of Type 2 Diabetes. *J. Clin. Endocrinol. Metab.* **2016**, *101*, 3212–3221. [CrossRef]

8. Rodríguez-Monforte, M.; Sánchez, E.; Barrio, F.; Costa, B.; Flores-Mateo, G. Metabolic Syndrome and Dietary Patterns: A Systematic Review and Meta-Analysis of Observational Studies. *Eur. J. Nutr.* **2017**, *56*, 925–947. [CrossRef]
9. Redruello-Requejo, M.; Samaniego-Vaesken, M.D.L.; Partearroyo, T.; Rodríguez-Alonso, P.; Soto-Méndez, M.J.; Hernández-Ruiz Á.; Villoslada, F.L.; Leis, R.; de Victoria, E.M.; Moreno, J.M.; et al. Dietary Intake of Individual (Intrinsic and Added) Sugars and Food Sources from Spanish Children Aged One to <10 Years-Results from the EsNuPI Study. *Nutrients* **2022**, *14*, 1667. [CrossRef]
10. Prinz, P. The Role of Dietary Sugars in Health: Molecular Composition or Just Calories? *Eur. J. Clin. Nutr.* **2019**, *73*, 1216–1223 [CrossRef]
11. Fidler Mis, N.; Braegger, C.; Bronsky, J.; Campoy, C.; Domellöf, M.; Embleton, N.D.; Hojsak, I.; Hulst, J.; Indrio, F.; Lapillonne, A.; et al. Sugar in Infants, Children and Adolescents: A Position Paper of the European Society for Paediatric Gastroenterology, Hepatology and Nutrition Committee on Nutrition. *J. Pediatr. Gastroenterol. Nutr.* **2017**, *65*, 681–696. [CrossRef]
12. Newens, K.J.; Walton, J. A Review of Sugar Consumption from Nationally Representative Dietary Surveys across the World. *J. Hum. Nutr. Diet.* **2016**, *29*, 225–240. [CrossRef] [PubMed]
13. Taskinen, M.R.; Packard, C.J.; Borén, J. Dietary Fructose and the Metabolic Syndrome. *Nutrients* **2019**, *11*, 1987. [CrossRef] [PubMed]
14. Malik, V.S.; Hu, F.B. Sugar-Sweetened Beverages and Cardiometabolic Health: An Update of the Evidence. *Nutrients* **2019**, *11*, 1840. [CrossRef] [PubMed]
15. Cox, C.L.; Stanhope, K.L.; Schwarz, J.M.; Graham, J.L.; Hatcher, B.; Griffen, S.C.; Bremer, A.A.; Berglund, L.; McGahan, J.P.; Keim, N.L.; et al. Circulating Concentrations of Monocyte Chemoattractant Protein-1, Plasminogen Activator Inhibitor-1, and Soluble Leukocyte Adhesion Molecule-1 in Overweight/Obese Men and Women Consuming Fructose- or Glucose-Sweetened Beverages for 10 Weeks. *J. Clin. Endocrinol. Metab.* **2011**, *96*, E2034–E2038. [CrossRef]
16. Della Corte, K.W.; Perrar, I.; Penczynski, K.J.; Schwingshackl, L.; Herder, C.; Buyken, A.E. Effect of Dietary Sugar Intake on Biomarkers of Subclinical Inflammation: A Systematic Review and Meta-Analysis of Intervention Studies. *Nutrients* **2018**, *10*, 606. [CrossRef]
17. Della Corte, K.A.; Penczynski, K.; Kuhnle, G.; Perrar, I.; Herder, C.; Roden, M.; Wudy, S.A.; Remer, T.; Alexy, U.; Buyken, A.E. The Prospective Association of Dietary Sugar Intake in Adolescence with Risk Markers of Type 2 Diabetes in Young Adulthood. *Front. Nutr.* **2021**, *7*, 362. [CrossRef]
18. Gill, J.M.R.; Sattar, N. Fruit Juice: Just Another Sugary Drink? *Lancet Diabetes Endocrinol.* **2014**, *2*, 444–446. [CrossRef]
19. Imamura, F.; O'Connor, L.; Ye, Z.; Mursu, J.; Hayashino, Y.; Bhupathiraju, S.N.; Forouhi, N.G. Consumption of Sugar Sweetened Beverages, Artificially Sweetened Beverages, and Fruit Juice and Incidence of Type 2 Diabetes: Systematic Review, Meta-Analysis, and Estimation of Population Attributable Fraction. *BMJ* **2015**, *351*, h3576. [CrossRef]
20. Choo, V.L.; Viguiliouk, E.; Blanco Mejia, S.; Cozma, A.I.; Khan, T.A.; Ha, V.; Wolever, T.M.S.; Leiter, L.A.; Vuksan, V.; Kendall, C.W.C.; et al. Food Sources of Fructose-Containing Sugars and Glycaemic Control: Systematic Review and Meta-Analysis of Controlled Intervention Studies. *BMJ* **2018**, *363*, k4644. [CrossRef]
21. Paglia, L. The Sweet Danger of Added Sugars. *Eur. J. Paediatr. Dent.* **2019**, *20*, 89. [CrossRef] [PubMed]
22. Spinelli, J.B.; Haigis, M.C. The Multifaceted Contributions of Mitochondria to Cellular Metabolism. *Nat. Cell Biol.* **2018**, *20*, 745. [CrossRef] [PubMed]
23. Pinti, M.v.; Fink, G.K.; Hathaway, Q.A.; Durr, A.J.; Kunovac, A.; Hollander, J.M.; Mv, P.; Gk, F.; Qa, H.; Aj, D.; et al. Mitochondrial dysfunction in type 2 diabetes mellitus: An organ-based analysis. *J. Physiol. Endocrinol. Metab.* **2019**, *316*, 268–285. [CrossRef] [PubMed]
24. Abdelmalek, M.F.; Suzuki, A.; Guy, C.; Unalp-Arida, A.; Colvin, R.; Johnson, R.J.; Diehl, A.M. Increased Fructose Consumption Is Associated with Fibrosis Severity in Patients with Nonalcoholic Fatty Liver Disease. *Hepatology* **2010**, *51*, 1961–1971. [CrossRef] [PubMed]
25. Sil, R.; Chakraborti, A.S. Oxidative Inactivation of Liver Mitochondria in High Fructose Diet-Induced Metabolic Syndrome in Rats: Effect of Glycyrrhizin Treatment. *Phytother. Res.* **2016**, *30*, 1503–1512. [CrossRef]
26. Grilo, L.F.; Tocantins, C.; Diniz, M.S.; Gomes, R.M.; Oliveira, P.J.; Matafome, P.; Pereira, S.P. Metabolic Disease Programming: From Mitochondria to Epigenetics, Glucocorticoid Signalling and Beyond. *Eur. J. Clin. Investig.* **2021**, *51*, e13625. [CrossRef]
27. Lou, P.H.; Lucchinetti, E.; Scott, K.Y.; Huang, Y.; Gandhi, M.; Hersberger, M.; Clanachan, A.S.; Lemieux, H.; Zaugg, M. Alterations in Fatty Acid Metabolism and Sirtuin Signaling Characterize Early Type-2 Diabetic Hearts of Fructose-Fed Rats. *Physiol. Rep.* **2017**, *5*, e13388. [CrossRef]
28. Zhang, Y.B.; Meng, Y.H.; Chang, S.; Zhang, R.Y.; Shi, C. High Fructose Causes Cardiac Hypertrophy via Mitochondrial Signaling Pathway. *Am. J. Transl. Res.* **2016**, *8*, 4869.
29. Szűcs, G.; Sója, A.; Péter, M.; Sárközy, M.; Bruszel, B.; Siska, A.; Földesi, I.; Szabó, Z.; Janáky, T.; Vígh, L.; et al. Prediabetes Induced by Fructose-Enriched Diet Influences Cardiac Lipidome and Proteome and Leads to Deterioration of Cardiac Function Prior to the Development of Excessive Oxidative Stress and Cell Damage. *Oxidative Med. Cell. Longev.* **2019**, *2019*, 3218275. [CrossRef]
30. García-Berumen, C.I.; Ortiz-Avila, O.; Vargas-Vargas, M.A.; del Rosario-Tamayo, B.A.; Guajardo-López, C.; Saavedra-Molina, A.; Rodríguez-Orozco, A.R.; Cortés-Rojo, C. The Severity of Rat Liver Injury by Fructose and High Fat Depends on the Degree of Respiratory Dysfunction and Oxidative Stress Induced in Mitochondria. *Lipids Health Dis.* **2019**, *18*, 78. [CrossRef]
31. Cioffi, F.; Senese, R.; Lasala, P.; Ziello, A.; Mazzoli, A.; Crescenzo, R.; Liverini, G.; Lanni, A.; Goglia, F.; Iossa, S. Fructose-Rich Diet Affects Mitochondrial DNA Damage and Repair in Rats. *Nutrients* **2017**, *9*, 323. [CrossRef] [PubMed]

32. Kannappan, S.; Palanisamy, N.; Anuradha, C.V. Suppression of Hepatic Oxidative Events and Regulation of ENOS Expression in the Liver by Naringenin in Fructose-Administered Rats. *Eur. J. Pharmacol.* **2010**, *645*, 177–184. [CrossRef] [PubMed]
33. Zaki, S.M.; Fattah, S.A.; Hassan, D.S. The Differential Effects of High-Fat and High-Fructose Diets on the Liver of Male Albino Rat and the Proposed Underlying Mechanisms. *Folia Morphol. (Warsz)* **2019**, *78*, 124–136. [CrossRef] [PubMed]
34. Beydogan, A.B.; Coskun, Z.M.; Bolkent, S. The Protective Effects of Δ9-Tetrahydrocannabinol against Inflammation and Oxidative Stress in Rat Liver with Fructose-Induced Hyperinsulinemia. *J. Pharm. Pharmacol.* **2019**, *71*, 408–416. [CrossRef] [PubMed]
35. Choi, Y.; Abdelmegeed, M.A.; Song, B.J. Diet High in Fructose Promotes Liver Steatosis and Hepatocyte Apoptosis in C57BL/6J Female Mice: Role of Disturbed Lipid Homeostasis and Increased Oxidative Stress. *Food Chem. Toxicol.* **2017**, *103*, 111–121. [CrossRef]
36. Cheng, S.M.; Cheng, Y.J.; Wu, L.Y.; Kuo, C.H.; Lee, Y.S.; Wu, M.C.; Huang, C.Y.; Ting, H.; Lee, S.-D. Activated Apoptotic and Anti-Survival Effects on Rat Hearts with Fructose Induced Metabolic Syndrome. *Cell Biochem. Funct.* **2014**, *32*, 133–141. [CrossRef]
37. Park, J.H.; Ku, H.J.; Kim, J.K.; Park, J.-W.; Lee, J.H. Amelioration of High Fructose-Induced Cardiac Hypertrophy by Naringin. *Sci. Rep.* **2018**, *8*, 9464. [CrossRef]
38. Kornfeld, O.S.; Qvit, N.; Haileselassie, B.; Shamloo, M.; Bernardi, P.; Mochly-Rosen, D. Interaction of Mitochondrial Fission Factor with Dynamin Related Protein 1 Governs Physiological Mitochondrial Function In Vivo. *Sci. Rep.* **2018**, *8*, 14034. [CrossRef]
39. Ihenacho, U.K.; Meacham, K.A.; Harwig, M.C.; Widlansky, M.E.; Hill, R.B. Mitochondrial Fission Protein 1: Emerging Roles in Organellar Form and Function in Health and Disease. *Front. Endocrinol. (Lausanne)* **2021**, *12*, 274. [CrossRef]
40. Suen, D.F.; Norris, K.L.; Youle, R.J. Mitochondrial Dynamics and Apoptosis. *Genes Dev.* **2008**, *22*, 1577–1590. [CrossRef]
41. Yu, T.; Sheu, S.S.; Robotham, J.L.; Yoon, Y. Mitochondrial Fission Mediates High Glucose-Induced Cell Death through Elevated Production of Reactive Oxygen Species. *Cardiovasc. Res.* **2008**, *79*, 341–351. [CrossRef] [PubMed]
42. Zheng, Y.; Luo, A.; Liu, X. The Imbalance of Mitochondrial Fusion/Fission Drives High-Glucose-Induced Vascular Injury. *Biomolecules* **2021**, *11*, 1779. [CrossRef] [PubMed]
43. Lee, W.C.; Chau, Y.Y.; Ng, H.Y.; Chen, C.H.; Wang, P.W.; Liou, C.W.; Lin, T.K.; Chen, J.B. Empagliflozin Protects HK-2 Cells from High Glucose-Mediated Injuries via a Mitochondrial Mechanism. *Cells* **2019**, *8*, 1085. [CrossRef]
44. Wang, X.; Yu, S.; Wang, C.Y.; Wang, Y.; Liu, H.X.; Cui, Y.; Zhang, L.-D. Advanced Glycation End Products Induce Oxidative Stress and Mitochondrial Dysfunction in SH-SY5Y Cells. *Vitr. Cell. Dev. Biol.-Anim.* **2015**, *51*, 204–209. [CrossRef] [PubMed]
45. Sung, S.K.; Woo, J.S.; Kim, Y.H.; Son, D.W.; Lee, S.W.; Song, G.S. Sildenafil Ameliorates Advanced Glycation End Products-Induced Mitochondrial Dysfunction in HT-22 Hippocampal Neuronal Cells. *J. Korean Neurosurg. Soc.* **2016**, *59*, 259–268. [CrossRef]
46. Ottum, M.S.; Mistry, A.M. Advanced Glycation End-Products: Modifiable Environmental Factors Profoundly Mediate Insulin Resistance. *J. Clin. Biochem. Nutr.* **2015**, *57*, 1–12. [CrossRef] [PubMed]
47. Singh, R.; Barden, A.; Mori, T.; Beilin, L. Advanced Glycation End-Products: A Review. *Diabetologia* **2001**, *44*, 129–146. [CrossRef]
48. Uribarri, J.; del Castillo, M.D.; de la Maza, M.P.; Filip, R.; Gugliucci, A.; Luevano-Contreras, C.; Macías-Cervantes, M.H.; Markowicz Bastos, D.H.; Medrano, A.; Menini, T.; et al. Dietary Advanced Glycation End Products and Their Role in Health and Disease. *Adv. Nutr.* **2015**, *6*, 461–473. [CrossRef]
49. Aragno, M.; Mastrocola, R. Dietary Sugars and Endogenous Formation of Advanced Glycation Endproducts: Emerging Mechanisms of Disease. *Nutrients* **2017**, *9*, 385. [CrossRef]
50. Yamagishi, S.; Matsui, T. Pathologic Role of Dietary Advanced Glycation End Products in Cardiometabolic Disorders, and Therapeutic Intervention. *Nutrition* **2016**, *32*, 157–165. [CrossRef]
51. Ruiz, H.H.; Ramasamy, R.; Schmidt, A.M. Advanced Glycation End Products: Building on the Concept of the "Common Soil" in Metabolic Disease. *Endocrinology* **2020**, *161*, bqz006. [CrossRef] [PubMed]
52. Jia, X.; Wu, L. Accumulation of Endogenous Methylglyoxal Impaired Insulin Signaling in Adipose Tissue of Fructose-Fed Rats. *Mol. Cell. Biochem.* **2007**, *306*, 133–139. [CrossRef] [PubMed]
53. Guo, Q.; Mori, T.; Jiang, Y.; Hu, C.; Osaki, Y.; Yoneki, Y.; Sun, Y.; Hosoya, T.; Kawamata, A.; Ogawa, S.; et al. Methylglyoxal Contributes to the Development of Insulin Resistance and Salt Sensitivity in Sprague Dawley Rats. *J. Hypertens.* **2009**, *27*, 1664–1671. [CrossRef] [PubMed]
54. Chen, J.; Jing, J.; Yu, S.; Song, M.; Tan, H.; Cui, B.; Huang, L. Advanced Glycation Endproducts Induce Apoptosis of Endothelial Progenitor Cells by Activating Receptor RAGE and NADPH Oxidase/JNK Signaling Axis. *Am. J. Transl. Res.* **2016**, *8*, 2169–2178.
55. Akhter, F.; Chen, D.; Akhter, A.; Sosunov, A.A.; Chen, A.; McKhann, G.M.; Yan, S.F.; Yan, S.S. High Dietary Advanced Glycation End Products Impair Mitochondrial and Cognitive Function. *J. Alzheimer's Dis.* **2020**, *76*, 165–178. [CrossRef]
56. Zhang, Y.; Huang, X.; Yuan, Y. Linagliptin Protects Human Chondrogenic ATDC5 Cells against Advanced Glycation End Products (AGEs)-Induced Apoptosis via a Mitochondria-Dependent Pathway. *Chem. Biol. Interact.* **2020**, *315*, 108901. [CrossRef]
57. Coughlan, M.T.; Yap, F.Y.T.; Tong, D.C.K.; Andrikopoulos, S.; Gasser, A.; Thallas-Bonke, V.; Webster, D.E.; Miyazaki, J.I.; Kay, T.W.; Slattery, R.M.; et al. Advanced Glycation End Products Are Direct Modulators of β-Cell Function. *Diabetes* **2011**, *60*, 2523–2532. [CrossRef]
58. Stephenson, J.; Heslehurst, N.; Hall, J.; Schoenaker, D.A.J.M.; Hutchinson, J.; Cade, J.E.; Poston, L.; Barrett, G.; Crozier, S.R.; Barker, M.; et al. Before the Beginning: Nutrition and Lifestyle in the Preconception Period and Its Importance for Future Health. *Lancet* **2018**, *391*, 1830–1841. [CrossRef]

59. Musial, B.; Vaughan, O.R.; Fernandez-Twinn, D.S.; Voshol, P.; Ozanne, S.E.; Fowden, A.L.; Sferruzzi-Perri, A.N. A Western-Style Obesogenic Diet Alters Maternal Metabolic Physiology with Consequences for Fetal Nutrient Acquisition in Mice. *J. Physiol.* **2017**, *595*, 4875–4892. [CrossRef]
60. Kereliuk, S.M.; Brawerman, G.M.; Dolinsky, V.W. Maternal Macronutrient Consumption and the Developmental Origins of Metabolic Disease in the Offspring. *Int. J. Mol. Sci.* **2017**, *18*, 1451. [CrossRef]
61. Grilo, L.F.; Diniz, M.S.; Tocantins, C.; Areia, A.L.; Pereira, S.P. The Endocrine–Metabolic Axis Regulation in Offspring Exposed to Maternal Obesity—Cause or Consequence in Metabolic Disease Programming? *Obesities* **2022**, *2*, 236–255. [CrossRef]
62. Cordero, P.; Vinciguerra, M.; Oben, J.A. *Maternal Perinatal Nutrition and Offspring Programming*; Elsevier Inc.: Amsterdam, The Netherlands, 2020; ISBN 9780128045725.
63. Barker, D.J.P. The Developmental Origins of Adult Disease. *J. Am. Coll. Nutr.* **2004**, *23*, 588S–595S. [CrossRef] [PubMed]
64. Lopes, G.A.D.; Ribeiro, V.L.B.; Barbisan, L.F.; Marchesan Rodrigues, M.A. Fetal Developmental Programing: Insights from Human Studies and Experimental Models. *J. Matern.-Fetal Neonatal Med.* **2017**, *30*, 722–728. [CrossRef] [PubMed]
65. Balakumar, M.; Raji, L.; Prabhu, D.; Sathishkumar, C.; Prabu, P.; Mohan, V.; Balasubramanyam, M. High-Fructose Diet Is as Detrimental as High-Fat Diet in the Induction of Insulin Resistance and Diabetes Mediated by Hepatic/Pancreatic Endoplasmic Reticulum (ER) Stress. *Mol. Cell. Biochem.* **2016**, *423*, 93–104. [CrossRef]
66. Saad, A.F.; Dickerson, J.; Kechichian, T.B.; Yin, H.; Gamble, P.; Salazar, A.; Patrikeev, I.; Motamedi, M.; Saade, G.R.; Costantine, M.M. High-Fructose Diet in Pregnancy Leads to Fetal Programming of Hypertension, Insulin Resistance, and Obesity in Adult Offspring. *Am. J. Obstet. Gynecol.* **2016**, *215*, 378.e1–378.e6. [CrossRef]
67. Toop, C.R.; Muhlhausler, B.S.; O'Dea, K.; Gentili, S. Impact of Perinatal Exposure to Sucrose or High Fructose Corn Syrup (HFCS-55) on Adiposity and Hepatic Lipid Composition in Rat Offspring. *J. Physiol.* **2017**, *595*, 4379–4398. [CrossRef]
68. Thompson, M.D.; Debosch, B.J. Maternal Fructose Diet-Induced Developmental Programming. *Nutrients* **2021**, *13*, 3278. [CrossRef]
69. Koo, S.; Kim, M.; Cho, H.M.; Kim, I. Maternal High-Fructose Intake during Pregnancy and Lactation Induces Metabolic Syndrome in Adult Offspring. *Nutr. Res. Pract.* **2021**, *15*, 160–172. [CrossRef]
70. Rodríguez, L.; Otero, P.; Panadero, M.I.; Rodrigo, S.; Álvarez-Millán, J.J.; Bocos, C. Maternal Fructose Intake Induces Insulin Resistance and Oxidative Stress in Male, but Not Female, Offspring. *J. Nutr. Metab.* **2015**, *2015*, 158091. [CrossRef]
71. Rodríguez, L.; Panadero, M.I.; Roglans, N.; Otero, P.; Rodrigo, S.; Álvarez-Millán, J.J.; Laguna, J.C.; Bocos, C. Fructose Only in Pregnancy Provokes Hyperinsulinemia, Hypoadiponectinemia, and Impaired Insulin Signaling in Adult Male, but Not Female, Progeny. *Eur. J. Nutr.* **2016**, *55*, 665–674. [CrossRef]
72. Clayton, Z.E.; Vickers, M.H.; Bernal, A.; Yap, C.; Sloboda, D.M. Early Life Exposure to Fructose Alters Maternal, Fetal and Neonatal Hepatic Gene Expression and Leads to Sex-Dependent Changes in Lipid Metabolism in Rat Offspring. *PLoS ONE* **2015**, *10*, e0141962. [CrossRef] [PubMed]
73. Mukai, Y.; Ozaki, H.; Serita, Y.; Sato, S. Maternal Fructose Intake during Pregnancy Modulates Hepatic and Hypothalamic AMP-Activated Protein Kinase Signalling in a Sex-Specific Manner in Offspring. *Clin. Exp. Pharmacol. Physiol.* **2014**, *41*, 331–337. [CrossRef] [PubMed]
74. Tain, Y.L.; Chan, J.Y.H.; Hsu, C.N. Maternal Fructose Intake Affects Transcriptome Changes and Programmed Hypertension in Offspring in Later Life. *Nutrients* **2016**, *8*, 757. [CrossRef] [PubMed]
75. Pascual, F.; Coleman, R.A. Fuel Availability and Fate in Cardiac Metabolism: A Tale of Two Substrates. *Biochim. Biophys. Acta Mol. Cell Biol. Lipids* **2016**, *1861*, 1425–1433. [CrossRef]
76. Leu, S.; Wu, K.L.H.; Lee, W.C.; Tain, Y.L.; Chan, J.Y.H. Maternal Fructose Intake Exacerbates Cardiac Remodeling in Offspring with Ventricular Pressure Overload. *Nutrients* **2021**, *13*, 3267. [CrossRef]
77. Torrealba, N.; Aranguiz, P.; Alonso, C.; Rothermel, B.A.; Lavandero, S. Mitochondria in Structural and Functional Cardiac Remodeling. *Adv. Exp. Med. Biol.* **2017**, *982*, 277–306. [CrossRef]
78. Mericq, V.; Piccardo, C.; Cai, W.; Chen, X.; Zhu, L.; Striker, G.E.; Vlassara, H.; Uribarri, J. Maternally Transmitted and Food-Derived Glycotoxins: A Factor Preconditioning the Young to Diabetes? *Diabetes Care* **2010**, *33*, 2232–2237. [CrossRef] [PubMed]
79. Gupta, A.; Uribarri, J. Dietary Advanced Glycation End Products and Their Potential Role in Cardiometabolic Disease in Children. *Horm. Res. Paediatr.* **2016**, *85*, 291–300. [CrossRef] [PubMed]
80. Csongová, M.; Gurecká, R.; Koborová, I.; Celec, P.; Domonkos, E.; Uličná, O.; Somoza, V.; Šebeková, K. The Effects of a Maternal Advanced Glycation End Product-Rich Diet on Somatic Features, Reflex Ontogeny and Metabolic Parameters of Offspring Mice. *Food Funct.* **2018**, *9*, 3432–3446. [CrossRef]
81. Francisco, F.A.; Barella, L.F.; Silveira, S.D.S.; Saavedra, L.P.J.; Prates, K.V.; Alves, V.S.; Franco, C.C.D.S.; Miranda, R.A.; Ribeiro, T.A.; Tófolo, L.P.; et al. Methylglyoxal Treatment in Lactating Mothers Leads to Type 2 Diabetes Phenotype in Male Rat Offspring at Adulthood. *Eur. J. Nutr.* **2018**, *57*, 477–486. [CrossRef]
82. Mortensen, O.H.; Larsen, L.H.; Ørstrup, L.K.H.; Hansen, L.H.L.; Grunnet, N.; Quistorff, B. Developmental Programming by High Fructose Decreases Phosphorylation Efficiency in Aging Offspring Brain Mitochondria, Correlating with Enhanced UCP5 Expression. *J. Cereb. Blood Flow Metab.* **2014**, *34*, 1205–1211. [CrossRef] [PubMed]
83. Yamada, H.; Munetsuna, E.; Yamazaki, M.; Mizuno, G.; Sadamoto, N.; Ando, Y.; Fujii, R.; Shiogama, K.; Ishikawa, H.; Suzuki, K.; et al. Maternal Fructose-Induced Oxidative Stress Occurs via Tfam and Ucp5 Epigenetic Regulation in Offspring Hippocampi. *FASEB J.* **2019**, *33*, 11431–11442. [CrossRef] [PubMed]

84. Bridges, H.R.; Jones, A.J.Y.; Pollak, M.N.; Hirst, J. Effects of Metformin and Other Biguanides on Oxidative Phosphorylation in Mitochondria. *Biochem. J.* **2014**, *462*, 475–487. [CrossRef] [PubMed]
85. Meng, Q.; Qi, X.; Fu, Y.; Chen, Q.; Cheng, P.; Yu, X.; Sun, X.; Wu, J.; Li, W.; Zhang, Q.; et al. Flavonoids Extracted from Mulberry (*Morus alba* L.) Leaf Improve Skeletal Muscle Mitochondrial Function by Activating AMPK in Type 2 Diabetes. *J. Ethnopharmacol.* **2020**, *248*, 112326. [CrossRef]
86. Gutierrez, J.A.; Liu, W.; Perez, S.; Xing, G.; Sonnenberg, G.; Kou, K.; Blatnik, M.; Allen, R.; Weng, Y.; Vera, N.B.; et al. Pharmacologic Inhibition of Ketohexokinase Prevents Fructose-Induced Metabolic Dysfunction. *Mol. Metab.* **2021**, *48*, 101196. [CrossRef]
87. van Poelje, P.D.; Potter, S.C.; Erion, M.D. Fructose-1, 6-Bisphosphatase Inhibitors for Reducing Excessive Endogenous Glucose Production in Type 2 Diabetes. *Handb. Exp. Pharmacol.* **2011**, *203*, 279–301. [CrossRef]
88. Mazzoli, A.; Spagnuolo, M.S.; Nazzaro, M.; Gatto, C.; Iossa, S.; Cigliano, L. Fructose Removal from the Diet Reverses Inflammation, Mitochondrial Dysfunction, and Oxidative Stress in Hippocampus. *Antioxidants* **2021**, *10*, 487. [CrossRef]
89. Huang, H.M.; Wu, C.W.; Chen, I.C.; Lee, Y.C.; Huang, Y.S.; Hung, C.Y.; Wu, K.L.H. Maternal High-Fructose Diet Induced Early-Onset Retinopathy via the Suppression of Synaptic Plasticity Mediated by Mitochondrial Dysfunction. *Am. J. Physiol. Endocrinol. Metab.* **2021**, *320*, E1173–E1182. [CrossRef]

diabetology

MDPI

Opinion

Impact of Dietary Sugars on β-Cell Function

Ananda Malta †, Lucas Paulo Jacinto Saavedra †, Scarlett Rodrigues Raposo, Gabriel Kian Guimarães Lopes, Maryana Debossan Fernandes, Letícia Ferreira Barbosa , Douglas Lopes Almeida and Paulo Cezar de Freitas Mathias *

Laboratory of Secretion Cell Biology, Department of Biotechnology, Genetics and Cell Biology, State University of Maringa, Maringá 87090-020, Brazil; nandamalt@hotmail.com (A.M.); saavedralpj@gmail.com (L.P.J.S.); scarlett_rr@hotmail.com (S.R.R.); dougalmeida84@gmail.com (D.L.A.)

* Correspondence: pcfmathias@gmail.com; Tel.: +55-4430114892

† These authors contributed equally to this work.

Abstract: Regular consumption of dietary sugars can cause significant damage to the β-cells. Almost a century after the discovery of insulin, it has been suggested that the frequent consumption of certain carbohydrates can damage pancreatic β-cells, causing disturbances in the regulation of insulin secretion. Most noncommunicable diseases, such as diabetes, obesity, and hypertension have a common origin, metabolic dysfunction, which is partly due to β-cell malfunction. In this article, we believed that sugars can lead to an imbalance in cellular metabolism, causing insulin exocytosis to dangerously increase or decrease blood insulin concentrations. In this study, we describe the major mechanism of insulin secretion and discuss the effects of sugar on pancreatic β-cells. Although many environmental factors strongly influence β-cells, occidental diet, including excess sugar, has been found to be the predominant factor that kills or disrupts the functioning of the unique cells that produce, store, and secrete insulin.

Keywords: pancreatic β-cell; insulin; diet; type 2 diabetes; sugar consumption

Citation: Malta, A.; Saavedra, L.P.J.; Raposo, S.R.; Lopes, G.K.G.; Fernandes, M.D.; Barbosa, L.F.; Almeida, D.L.; Mathias, P.C.d.F. Impact of Dietary Sugars on β-Cell Function. *Diabetology* **2023**, *4*, 178–183. https://doi.org/10.3390/diabetology4020017

Academic Editor: Yoshifumi Saisho

Received: 4 April 2023
Revised: 22 April 2023
Accepted: 23 April 2023
Published: 1 May 2023

1. Introduction

The previous year marked 100 years since the discovery of insulin, a drug responsible for saving and mitigating the sufferings of millions diagnosed with diabetes mellitus (DM). DM is characterized by the dyshomeostasis of glucose metabolism, which leads to a chronic increase in blood glucose levels, primarily due to insulin secretion dysfunction and/or impaired insulin action in peripheral tissues [1,2]. Excessive consumption of added sugars, mainly fructose and sucrose, is highly correlated with DM, which can lead to insulin resistance, not only in adults [3] but also in children and young people [4].

The purpose of this opinion article is to highlight the current available literature on DM and discuss the impact of dietary sugars on pancreatic β-cells and diabetes development.

2. Endocrine Pancreas

Insulin is a hormone capable of decreasing blood glucose levels. It is produced, stored, and secreted by β-cells of the Langerhans islets in the pancreas. Each islet contains different types of endocrine cells. Insulin-secreting β-cells are the most abundant cell type (~80%) in the islets, followed by pancreatic α-cells (~15%) that secrete the hormone glucagon, and pancreatic δ-cells (5%) that secrete somatostatin, along with a small number of PP cells secreting pancreatic polypeptide. Endocrine cells account for <1% of the pancreatic tissue, while the rest are composed of exocrine cells, which produce digestive juices containing enzymes, such as proteases, lipases, and amylases; exocrine cells are responsible for degrading meal components, including carbohydrates, into the gut [5,6]. Functional pancreatic endocrine development occurs during gestation and continues until infancy. Specifically, β-cells can remodel or proliferate during the early postnatal period; however, the number of these cells remains constant for the rest of life. Thus, destruction or malfunction of β-cells can lead to drastic metabolic dysfunction, causing DM [7].

3. β-Cells Burn Sugar to Provide Fuel to other Cells

Pancreatic β-cells can be considered metabolic sensors presenting a stimulus-secretion coupling with metabolism, including carbohydrate degradation. Glucose is the major hexose derived from carbohydrate-rich meals. Pancreatic β-cells capture glucose by specific transporters, such as glucose transport proteins (GLUT-2), located in the plasma membrane. Similar to other cells, β-cells degrade all six carbon atoms of glucose and convert the energy contained in their molecules into a small metabolite, adenosine triphosphate (ATP). Similar to neurons, β-cells are electrically excited. When depolarized, β-cells change their architecture and functions. Immediately after ATP production, β-cells are depolarized and a sequence of intracellular events occurs, culminating in the exocytosis of insulin in the blood. Specifically, by increasing the ATP/ADP ratio, ATP inhibits the activity of ATP-dependent potassium ($K^{+}{}_{ATP}$) channels, which drive K^+ ions into the extracellular medium via gradient straining. Subsequently, K^+ ions are trapped in the cytosol, which increases the positive cell charge. In this case, depolarization enhances the activity of certain calcium (Ca^{2+}) channels, thereby promoting the influx of Ca^{2+} from the extracellular medium. The free intracellular Ca^{2+} concentration increases and activates proteins that stimulate the cytoskeleton to transport insulin vesicles to the periphery of the cell membrane, leading to exocytosis. Together, these mechanisms are known as the "fuel hypothesis" that leads to insulin stimulus-secretion coupling, where nutrients act as a fuel to induce insulin secretion in pancreatic β-cells (Figure 1) [8].

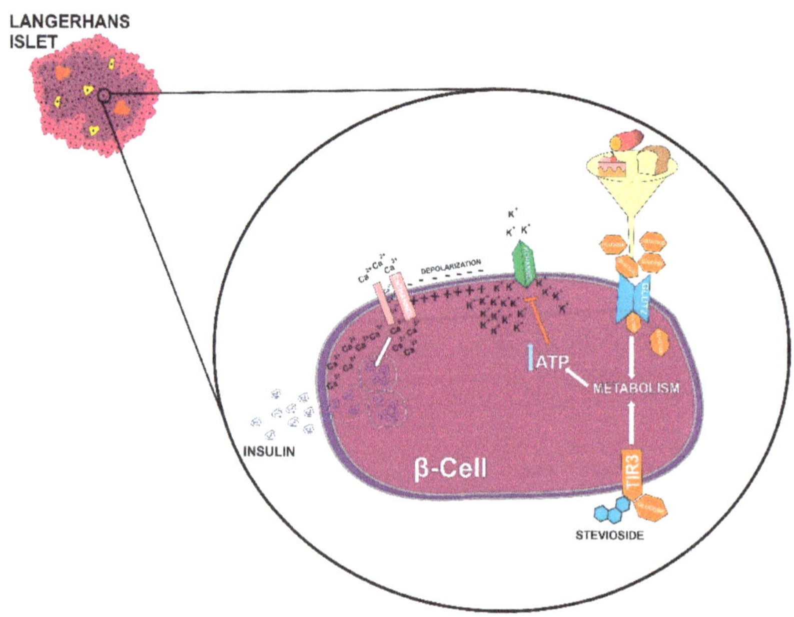

Figure 1. Glucose is transported to the β-cell mediated by the Glut2 membrane transporter. The intracellular metabolism of glucose induces changes in electrical activity, which culminate in an increase in the cytoplasmic Ca^{2+} concentration and exocytosis of insulin granules. The sweet taste receptor TIR3 is expressed in the pancreatic β-cells and is activated by various sugars, including sucrose, fructose, and glucose, and artificial sweeteners, such as stevioside, stimulating insulin secretion by increasing the metabolism of nutrients to produce ATP.

4. Great Conflict: Fuel Hypothesis vs. Glucose Receptor

In spite of the fuel insulin secretion-coupling, glucose stimulates insulin secretion in pancreatic β-cells, despite maintaining potassium-ATP channels under lowered activities, indicating an alternative pathway as a mechanism for glucose and other fuel metabolites to amplify their stimulation via ATP. This alternative mechanism can also be observed in neurotransmitters, such as acetylcholine, which bind to plasma membrane receptors and mediate an increase in intracellular Ca^{2+} levels and the ability of activated protein kinase C to increase the efficiency of Ca^{2+} in insulin exocytosis [8,9]. Therefore, glucose acts as the primary nutrient stimulating insulin secretion. Other nutrients, amino acids, and free fatty acids are capable of increasing insulin secretion, mostly through mechanisms involving the fuel hypothesis; however, the presence of glucose is required for them to be effective.

Numerous other hexoses and other monosaccharides, heptoses, pentoses, tetroses and trioses, aldoses or ketoses, or conjugated glucosamine can directly stimulate β-cells, coupling insulin secretion to energy transformation using carbohydrates as a nutrient; however, some of them, such as fructose and mannoheptulose, have demonstrated no or a weak capacity [10,11]. The fuel hypothesis was initially based on an artificial leucine, 2-amino-bicycle (2,2,1) heptane-2-carboxylic acid, which does not break down; however, it stimulates the metabolism of cells to produce ATP and induces insulin secretion [12].

Four decades of evidence collected through clinical and experimental trials support the idea of stimulus secretion-coupling for the metabolism of pancreatic β-cells. A recently proposed idea suggests that β-cells are equipped with receptors for glucose or nutrient secretagogues, such as monosaccharides, amino acids, and free fatty acids; however, these receptors have not yet been isolated. Despite this complex controversy, it has been shown to be a receptor for sweetness in the β-cell membranes.

5. β-Cells Sense Sweet, Bitter, Umami, and Salty Taste

Natural sweeteners, such as glucose and fructose, or artificial sweeteners with no caloric value, such as some fractions from *Stevia rabaudiana bertonni* leaves, sucralose extracted from sugar cane, aspartame from laboratory synthesis of amino acids, and cyclamate and saccharin obtained from petroleum, can bind to β-cell sweet taste receptors. The heterodimer comprises two members of the class C G protein-coupled receptor: type 1 taste receptor-2 (T1R2) and T1R3 (the dominant subunit expressed in pancreatic islets) [13–18]. Once sweeteners bind, they target a response to accelerate the degradation of stored nutrients, such as glucose, amino acids, and free fatty acids, to produce ATP and stimulate insulin granule exocytosis (Figure 1) [19].

6. Sugar Sources Potentially Transport Poisons or Medicines to β-Cells

The occidental diet is rich in glucose and fructose, which are the major sources of carbohydrates from different mono-and/or polysaccharides such as sucrose, starch, and sugar from other farinaceous foods. Most of these are processed by industries, eliminating other macro- and micro-compounds, fibers, and vitamins. High level daily consumption of carbohydrate sources can compromise the β-cells [20]. β-cells can be killed or become dysfunctional due to glucotoxicity, leading to type 2 diabetes (non-insulin-dependent) [21]. The impact of different sources of monosaccharides on β-cell function can be dependent on the amount consumed, carbohydrate source type, and environment. In some countries, there is a massive intake of fructose-rich corn syrup. This carbohydrate is captured less by β-cell, contrasting with hepatic cells. Most fructose metabolism occurs in the liver, and its excess causes hepatic dysfunction, which indirectly perturbs β-cell function through high glucose production and hepatic fat dysfunction [22]. Other sources of carbohydrates, such as manioca or sweet potato, and other vegetables and fruits rich in natural fiber, are less dangerous to β-cells [23]. Fibers stimulate intestinal contraction and increase intestinal transit, which reduces monosaccharide absorption, thus helping in glycemia attenuation [24,25]. One important effect of these sugar sources is the reduced insulin secretion from β-cells, which does not demand an increased amount of circulating insulin to maintain low glycemia. Under these conditions, cells are protected from glucotoxicity. In contrast, diets with low fiber are associated with an increased risk of type 2 diabetes, which has been observed in women with a sedentary lifestyle and family history of diabetes [26]

Apart from fibers, fruits and artificial sweeteners also contain antioxidants, which can help protect β-cell function [27,28]. However, sugars with a high reducing capacity, such as ribose and fructose, can suppress insulin gene transcription and provoke oxidative stress-inducing apoptosis of β-cells [29].

7. Environment as Vectorial to β-Cell

Although we discuss β-cell function and focus on the mechanisms of insulin secretion stimulated by carbohydrates, it is important to consider the myriad of biological factors. Pre-and postprandial time durations have the potential to stimulate, potentiate, or inhibit insulin secretion processes. Any pancreatic β-cell dysfunction combined with high carbohydrate consumption can compromise entire metabolic regulation and provoke cardiometabolic diseases, such as obesity, diabetes, and hypertension [30].

The autonomic nervous system controls β-cell function. Under normal physiological situations of meal intake, the parasympathetic nervous system (PNS) potentiates glucose-insulin secretion coupling, whereas the sympathetic nervous system (SNS) inhibits it [31,32]. This is an equilibrium action; however, an imbalance may occur, as in obesity, where PNS is enhanced and SNS is decreased. Under these conditions β-cells oversecrete insulin, which causes fasting hyperinsulinemia, tissue insulin resistance, and high hepatic glucose production leading to excess blood glucose concentrations; thus, excessive carbohydrate consumption can aggravate metabolic dysfunction [33,34].

The central nervous system directly regulates insulin secretion. Recently, it was shown that the paraventricular hypothalamic nucleus (PVN), when stimulated immediately, suppresses the insulin secretion process via SNS neurons connected to β-cell; conversely, low blood glucose concentration is detected by the PVN, which allows rapid increase of glucose-induced insulin secretion. High sugar intake disrupts the central control of insulin secretion, causing cardiometabolic dysfunction [35,36].

Exercise is another important factor. Physical training improves the peripheral tissue insulin sensitivity, which reduces the demand for insulin secretion. Exercise also induces irisin from the muscle, which directly potentiates glucose-induced insulin secretion from β-cells; however, even physically trained individuals consuming calorie-dense diets can develop β-cell malfunction [37,38].

Additionally, overconsumption of fructose affects the gut microbiota. The gut microbiota consists of numerous gastrointestinal microorganisms. Diet, including the carbohydrate source and their quantities, can determine microbiota composition. High fructose consumption causes dysbiosis of the microbiota, which leads to increased gut barrier permeability, inflammation, and the progression of metabolic diseases [39].

Since the 18th century industrial revolution, the environment has changed considerably, ultimately compromising the health of human beings as well as that of animals and plants. Air, water, and food sources contain acids, heavy metals, plastics, and radiation, among many other poisons, that have the ability to disrupt metabolism, causing cardiometabolic dysfunction [40]. The β-cells are also a target for contaminants that combine with occidental diet increasing the risk of disrupting the insulin secretion process [41].

8. Conclusions and Future Perspectives

Considering that β-cells are a highly sensible target in many stressful situations, they exert their effects in a combined manner. Thus, it can be concluded that it is difficult to analyze the impact of different carbohydrate sources on pancreatic β-cells.

Given the delicate nature of β-cells as an "organ", numerous studies have suggested changes in the occidental diet to reduce the exposure of certain carbohydrates to the β-cells.

Author Contributions: Conceptualization and Methodology, A.M., L.P.J.S. and P.C.d.F.M. Writing—Original Draft Preparation, A.M., L.P.J.S. and P.C.d.F.M.; S.R.R., M.D.F., D.L.A., G.K.G.L., L.F.B.: Writing—Review & Editing. All authors have read and agreed to the published version of the manuscript.

Funding: Brazilian Federal Foundation, Conselho Nacional de Desenvolvimento Científico e Tecnológico (CNPq), Coordenação de Aperfeiçoamento de Pessoal de Nível Superior (CAPES), and Group JBS.

Institutional Review Board Statement: Not applicable.

Informed Consent Statement: Not applicable.

Data Availability Statement: Not applicable.

Conflicts of Interest: The authors declare no conflict of interest. The funders had no role in the study design; collection, analyses, or interpretation of data; writing of the manuscript; or decision to publish the results.

References

1. Ashcroft, F.M.; Rorsman, P. Diabetes mellitus and the beta cell: The last ten years. *Cell* **2012**, *148*, 1160–1171. [CrossRef]
2. Eizirik, D.L.; Pasquali, L.; Cnop, M. Pancreatic beta-cells in type 1 and type 2 diabetes mellitus: Different pathways to failure. *Nat. Rev. Endocrinol.* **2020**, *16*, 349–362. [CrossRef] [PubMed]
3. McKeown, N.M.; Meigs, J.B.; Liu, S.; Saltzman, E.; Wilson, P.W.; Jacques, P.F. Carbohydrate nutrition, insulin resistance, and the prevalence of the metabolic syndrome in the Framingham Offspring Cohort. *Diabetes Care* **2004**, *27*, 538–546. [CrossRef] [PubMed]
4. Davis, J.N.; Ventura, E.E.; Weigensberg, M.J.; Ball, G.D.; Cruz, M.L.; Shaibi, G.Q.; Goran, M.I. The relation of sugar intake to beta cell function in overweight Latino children. *Am. J. Clin. Nutr.* **2005**, *82*, 1004–1010. [CrossRef] [PubMed]
5. MacDonald, P.E.; Rorsman, P. Oscillations, intercellular coupling, and insulin secretion in pancreatic beta cells. *PLoS Biol.* **2006**, *4*, e49. [CrossRef]
6. Bock, T.; Pakkenberg, B.; Buschard, K. Genetic background determines the size and structure of the endocrine pancreas. *Diabetes* **2005**, *54*, 133–137. [CrossRef] [PubMed]
7. Cnop, M.; Welsh, N.; Jonas, J.C.; Jorns, A.; Lenzen, S.; Eizirik, D.L. Mechanisms of pancreatic beta-cell death in type 1 and type 2 diabetes: Many differences, few similarities. *Diabetes* **2005**, *54* (Suppl. 2), S97–S107. [CrossRef] [PubMed]
8. Rorsman, P.; Ashcroft, F.M. Pancreatic Beta-Cell Electrical Activity and Insulin Secretion: Of Mice and Men. *Physiol. Rev.* **2018**, *98*, 117–214. [CrossRef]
9. Mourad, N.I.; Nenquin, M.; Henquin, J.C. Metabolic amplifying pathway increases both phases of insulin secretion independently of beta-cell actin microfilaments. *Am. J. Physiol. Cell Physiol.* **2010**, *299*, C389–C398. [CrossRef]
10. Teraoku, H.; Lenzen, S. Dynamics of Insulin Secretion from EndoC-betaH1 beta-Cell Pseudoislets in Response to Glucose and Other Nutrient and Nonnutrient Secretagogues. *J. Diabetes Res.* **2017**, *2017*, 2309630. [CrossRef]
11. Curry, D.L. Effects of mannose and fructose on the synthesis and secretion of insulin. *Pancreas* **1989**, *4*, 2–9. [CrossRef] [PubMed]
12. Sener, A.; Malaisse, W.J. L-leucine and a nonmetabolized analogue activate pancreatic islet glutamate dehydrogenase. *Nature* **1980**, *288*, 187–189. [CrossRef]
13. Malaisse, W.J. Insulin release: The receptor hypothesis. *Diabetologia* **2014**, *57*, 1287–1290. [CrossRef] [PubMed]
14. von Molitor, E.; Riedel, K.; Krohn, M.; Rudolf, R.; Hafner, M.; Cesetti, T. An alternative pathway for sweet sensation: Possible mechanisms and physiological relevance. *Pflugers Arch.* **2020**, *472*, 1667–1691. [CrossRef]
15. Abudula, R.; Jeppesen, P.B.; Rolfsen, S.E.; Xiao, J.; Hermansen, K. Rebaudioside A potently stimulates insulin secretion from isolated mouse islets: Studies on the dose-, glucose-, and calcium-dependency. *Metabolism* **2004**, *53*, 1378–1381. [CrossRef] [PubMed]
16. Philippaert, K.; Pironet, A.; Mesuere, M.; Sones, W.; Vermeiren, L.; Kerselaers, S.; Pinto, S.; Segal, A.; Antoine, N.; Gysemans, C.; et al. Steviol glycosides enhance pancreatic beta-cell function and taste sensation by potentiation of TRPM5 channel activity. *Nat. Commun.* **2017**, *8*, 14733. [CrossRef] [PubMed]
17. Kyriazis, G.A.; Soundarapandian, M.M.; Tyrberg, B. Sweet taste receptor signaling in beta cells mediates fructose-induced potentiation of glucose-stimulated insulin secretion. *Proc. Natl. Acad. Sci. USA* **2012**, *109*, E524–E532. [CrossRef]
18. Malaisse, W.J.; Vanonderbergen, A.; Louchami, K.; Jijakli, H.; Malaisse-Lagae, F. Effects of artificial sweeteners on insulin release and cationic fluxes in rat pancreatic islets. *Cell Signal.* **1998**, *10*, 727–733. [CrossRef]
19. Nakagawa, Y.; Nagasawa, M.; Yamada, S.; Hara, A.; Mogami, H.; Nikolaev, V.O.; Lohse, M.J.; Shigemura, N.; Ninomiya, Y.; Kojima, I. Sweet taste receptor expressed in pancreatic beta-cells activates the calcium and cyclic AMP signaling systems and stimulates insulin secretion. *PLoS ONE* **2009**, *4*, e5106. [CrossRef]
20. Alam, Y.H.; Kim, R.; Jang, C. Metabolism and Health Impacts of Dietary Sugars. *J. Lipid Atheroscler.* **2022**, *11*, 20–38. [CrossRef]

21. Oberhauser, L.; Jimenez-Sanchez, C.; Madsen, J.G.S.; Duhamel, D.; Mandrup, S.; Brun, T.; Maechler, P. Glucolipotoxicity promotes the capacity of the glycerolipid/NEFA cycle supporting the secretory response of pancreatic beta cells. *Diabetologia* **2022**, *65*, 705–720. [CrossRef]
22. Rizkalla, S.W. Health implications of fructose consumption: A review of recent data. *Nutr. Metab.* **2010**, *7*, 82. [CrossRef]
23. Chandrasekara, A.; Josheph Kumar, T. Roots and Tuber Crops as Functional Foods: A Review on Phytochemical Constituents and Their Potential Health Benefits. *Int. J. Food Sci.* **2016**, *2016*, 3631647. [CrossRef]
24. Cherbut, C.; Bruley des Varannes, S.; Schnee, M.; Rival, M.; Galmiche, J.P.; Delort-Laval, J. Involvement of small intestinal motility in blood glucose response to dietary fibre in man. *Br. J. Nutr.* **1994**, *71*, 675–685. [CrossRef]
25. Lattimer, J.M.; Haub, M.D. Effects of dietary fiber and its components on metabolic health. *Nutrients* **2010**, *2*, 1266–1289. [CrossRef]
26. Schulze, M.B.; Liu, S.; Rimm, E.B.; Manson, J.E.; Willett, W.C.; Hu, F.B. Glycemic index, glycemic load, and dietary fiber intake and incidence of type 2 diabetes in younger and middle-aged women. *Am. J. Clin. Nutr.* **2004**, *80*, 348–356. [CrossRef]
27. Chattopadhyay, S.; Raychaudhuri, U.; Chakraborty, R. Artificial sweeteners—A review. *J. Food Sci. Technol.* **2014**, *51*, 611–621. [CrossRef] [PubMed]
28. Lourenco, S.C.; Moldao-Martins, M.; Alves, V.D. Antioxidants of Natural Plant Origins: From Sources to Food Industry Applications. *Molecules* **2019**, *24*, 4132. [CrossRef]
29. Matsuoka, T.; Kajimoto, Y.; Watada, H.; Kaneto, H.; Kishimoto, M.; Umayahara, Y.; Fujitani, Y.; Kamada, T.; Kawamori, R.; Yamasaki, Y. Glycation-dependent, reactive oxygen species-mediated suppression of the insulin gene promoter activity in HIT cells. *J. Clin. Investig.* **1997**, *99*, 144–150. [CrossRef] [PubMed]
30. Wali, J.A.; Raubenheimer, D.; Senior, A.M.; Le Couteur, D.G.; Simpson, S.J. Cardio-metabolic consequences of dietary carbohydrates: Reconciling contradictions using nutritional geometry. *Cardiovasc. Res.* **2021**, *117*, 386–401. [CrossRef] [PubMed]
31. Gautam, D.; Han, S.J.; Hamdan, F.F.; Jeon, J.; Li, B.; Li, J.H.; Cui, Y.; Mears, D.; Lu, H.; Deng, C.; et al. A critical role for beta cell M3 muscarinic acetylcholine receptors in regulating insulin release and blood glucose homeostasis in vivo. *Cell Metab.* **2006**, *3*, 449–461. [CrossRef]
32. Lundquist, I.; Ericson, L.E. beta-Adrenergic insulin release and adrenergic innervation of mouse pancreatic islets. *Cell Tissue Res.* **1978**, *193*, 73–85. [CrossRef]
33. Bray, G.A. Obesity, a disorder of nutrient partitioning: The MONA LISA hypothesis. *J. Nutr.* **1991**, *121*, 1146–1162. [CrossRef]
34. Vozarova de Courten, B.; Weyer, C.; Stefan, N.; Horton, M.; DelParigi, A.; Havel, P.; Bogardus, C.; Tataranni, P.A. Parasympathetic blockade attenuates augmented pancreatic polypeptide but not insulin secretion in Pima Indians. *Diabetes* **2004**, *53*, 663–671. [CrossRef] [PubMed]
35. Papazoglou, I.; Lee, J.H.; Cui, Z.; Li, C.; Fulgenzi, G.; Bahn, Y.J.; Staniszewska-Goraczniak, H.M.; Pinol, R.A.; Hogue, I.B.; Enquist, L.W.; et al. A distinct hypothalamus-to-beta cell circuit modulates insulin secretion. *Cell Metab.* **2022**, *34*, 285–298.e7. [CrossRef]
36. Gaur, A.; Pal, G.K.; Pal, P. Role of Ventromedial Hypothalamus in Sucrose-Induced Obesity on Metabolic Parameters. *Ann. Neurosci* **2021**, *28*, 39–46. [CrossRef]
37. Zhu, W.; Sahar, N.E.; Javaid, H.M.A.; Pak, E.S.; Liang, G.; Wang, Y.; Ha, H.; Huh, J.Y. Exercise-Induced Irisin Decreases Inflammation and Improves NAFLD by Competitive Binding with MD2. *Cells* **2021**, *10*, 3306. [CrossRef] [PubMed]
38. Zheng, S.; Chen, N.; Kang, X.; Hu, Y.; Shi, S. Irisin alleviates FFA induced beta-cell insulin resistance and inflammatory response through activating PI3K/AKT/FOXO1 signaling pathway. *Endocrine* **2021**, *75*, 740–751. [CrossRef] [PubMed]
39. Cheng, W.L.; Li, S.J.; Lee, T.I.; Lee, T.W.; Chung, C.C.; Kao, Y.H.; Chen, Y.J. Sugar Fructose Triggers Gut Dysbiosis and Metabolic Inflammation with Cardiac Arrhythmogenesis. *Biomedicines* **2021**, *9*, 728. [CrossRef]
40. Almeida, D.L.; Pavanello, A.; Saavedra, L.P.; Pereira, T.S.; de Castro-Prado, M.A.A.; de Freitas Mathias, P.C. Environmental monitoring and the developmental origins of health and disease. *J. Dev. Orig. Health Dis.* **2019**, *10*, 608–615. [CrossRef]
41. Fabricio, G.; Malta, A.; Chango, A.; De Freitas Mathias, P.C. Environmental Contaminants and Pancreatic Beta-Cells. *J. Clin. Res. Pediatr. Endocrinol.* **2016**, *8*, 257–263. [CrossRef] [PubMed]

diabetology

MDPI

Review

Impact of Sugars on Hypothalamic Satiety Pathways and Its Contribution to Dysmetabolic States

Adriana M. Capucho and Silvia V. Conde *

NOVA Medical School, Faculdade de Ciências Médicas, Universidade NOVA de Lisboa, Rua Câmara Pestana 6, Edifício 2, piso 3, 1150-082 Lisboa, Portugal
* Correspondence: silvia.conde@nms.unl.pt

Abstract: Food behaviour is a complex and multifaceted cooperation between physiologic, psychological, social, and genetic factors, influencing meal timing, amount of food intake, food preferences, and food selections. Deregulation of the neurobiological mechanisms controlling food behaviour underlies the development of obesity and type 2 diabetes, two epidemics of the present century. Several brain nuclei are involved in the regulation of the different components of food behaviours; the hypothalamus is the key in controlling appetite and energy homeostasis. In this review, we will explain the role of the hypothalamus in the control of food intake and its interplay with other brain nuclei important in food behaviour. We will also highlight the deregulation of satiety pathways in type 2 diabetes and obesity and the mechanisms behind this deregulation. Finally, knowing that there are different categories of sugars and that they differently impact food behaviours, we will review in a concise manner the studies referring to the effects of sugars in satiety and reward pathways and their impacts on metabolic diseases.

Keywords: hypothalamus; hypercaloric diets; sugar; satiety pathways; diabetes

Citation: Capucho, A.M.; Conde, S.V. Impact of Sugars on Hypothalamic Satiety Pathways and Its Contribution to Dysmetabolic States. *Diabetology* **2023**, *4*, 1–10. https://doi.org/10.3390/diabetology4010001

Academic Editor: Jang Hyun Choi

Received: 23 November 2022
Revised: 9 December 2022
Accepted: 15 December 2022
Published: 24 December 2022

1. Introduction

In the last decades, we have witnessed an escalating number of individuals suffering from metabolic diseases, such as obesity, and its associated diseases, such as metabolic syndrome and type 2 diabetes (T2D). These metabolic diseases are genetic conditions [1] that are mainly associated with modern lifestyles; they are characterised by physical inactivity, sedentarism, and hypercaloric diets [1,2]. While obesity affects 650 million people worldwide, it is estimated that 463 million people between the ages of 20 and 79 suffer from diabetes, representing 9.3% of the world's population within this age range. In 2030, it is estimated that this number will rise to 578 million people (10.2%) and 700 million (10.9%) in 2045. What is even more worrying is that in 2019, globally, an estimated 4.2 million people died from diabetes and its complications [3]. Diabetes is a chronic metabolic condition characterised by high blood glucose levels due to the inability of the body to produce enough insulin to reduce glucose levels and due to the inefficiency of insulin, a phenomenon designated as insulin resistance [4,5]. T2D, a diabetes condition, typically begins with the development of insulin resistance. During this period, pancreatic β-cells are stimulated to increase insulin production and secreted to maintain normal blood glucose concentration. Upon diagnosis of T2D, approximately 40–50% of the β-cells are already dysfunctional and no longer able to compensate for the high levels of circulating glucose. This phenomenon results in glucose intolerance, which ultimately leads to a state of fasting hyperglycaemia [4,6]. Obesity is an established risk factor in the development of T2D, resulting from the deregulation of energy metabolism, which is also crucial in the control of T2D. The central nervous system (CNS) and, in particular, the hypothalamus, plays a crucial role in the control of energy homeostasis since it regulates functions, such as satiety and thermogenesis [7]. These functions are known to be altered in states of dysmetabolism; therefore, they play an important role in the setting and maintenance of metabolic diseases.

This manuscript focuses on and summarises the importance of the hypothalamus in the control of satiety pathways and its role in dysmetabolic states, particularly in T2D and obesity. In addition, we review the impact of sugar consumption on satiety pathways and reward systems in the development of T2D.

2. Control of Food Intake by the Hypothalamus

Food behaviour is a complex coordination of physiologic, psychological, social, and genetic factors influencing meal timing, the quantity of food intake, food preference, and food selection. It is regulated by several different brain circuits, where the hypothalamus is essential in controlling appetite and energy homeostasis. The hypothalamus is located below the thalamus near the pituitary gland, above the brainstem [8]. The first insight into the key role of the hypothalamus in food intake came from the observation that humans and animals with lesions in the hypothalamus brain region showed a rapid onset of obesity [9]. In fact, when the ventromedial hypothalamic nuclei (VMH) were lesioned with electrical current, the rats exhibited increased food intake and adiposity [10] Afterward, in the 1950s, Delgado and Anand examined the effects of lesions in the VMH in cats by applying chronic (5–10 days) electrostimulation in this region; they observed an increase in food intake [11]. Of importance, the authors performed the same lesions in another hypothalamic nucleus with the same parameters, but this did not produce similar effects [11]. This nucleus is known as the "satiety center" [12]. Apart from the VMH, the lateral hypothalamic area (LHA) is also known to play a key role in the regulation of ingestive behaviour (ever since the early studies on lesions conducted by Anand and Brobeck, where they found that bilateral electrolytic lesions of LHA completely inhibited food intake to the point where the rat died of starvation) [13]. In fact, LHA is called the "feeding center" [14]. Ono et al. [15] showed later that LHA is also involved in functions associated with rewards, emotions, aversion, and learning. Although these two hypothalamic nuclei are very important in the control of food intake, the arcuate nucleus (ARC) is critical to the regulation of food intake and energy metabolism (Figure 1). The ARC has a perfect location near the median eminence (ME) that is rich in fenestrated capillaries receiving information from the blood–brain barrier. The ME plays a role in the transport of hormonal and nutritional signals from the periphery to the hypothalamus [7]. These signals are sensed by two antagonistic types of neurons: (1) the neuropeptide Y (NPY)-agouti-related peptide (AgRP)-expressing neurons (AgRP/NPY neurons), also called orexigenic neurons or appetite-stimulating neurons and; (2) the pro-opiomelanocortin (POMC) and cocaine- and amphetamine-regulated transcript (CART) neurons (POMC/CART neurons), called anorexigenic neurons/appetite-suppressing neurons. These neurons exhibit receptors for hormones, such as leptin, insulin, and glucagon-like peptide 1 (GLP-1), which regulate satiety, glucose homeostasis, insulin signalling, and energy expenditure [7,16] (Figure 1). In the POMC/CART neurons, these substances promote satiety, while in the AgRP/NPY neurons, they act antagonistically to inhibit these neurons, therefore reducing appetite and increasing energy expenditure. The POMC/CART neurons mainly project to second-order neurons in the paraventricular nucleus (PVN), but also to another hypothalamic nucleus, such as the VMH, dorsomedial hypothalamus (DMH), and the LHA. These second-order neurons have an important role in processing the received information from the ARC, projecting to other brain regions to trigger a response to maintain energy homeostasis. After food injection, POMC is cleaved to the α-melanocyte-stimulating hormone (α-MSH) that binds to melanocortin 3 and 4 receptor (MC3/4R) neurons in the ARC and PVN (Figure 1). Several studies reported that food intake is inhibited by hypothalamic MC4R neurons in a constant manner [17] and that MC4R activation, mainly in the PVN, leads to an increase in energy expenditure by triggering the sympathetic nervous system activation, particularly in the brown adipose tissue (BAT) [18,19]. This important role of MC4R receptors in the regulation of food behaviour and energy homeostasis is confirmed by the presence of a severe obesity phenotype in MC4R-deficient subjects [20] and by the use of MC4R agonists, such as setmelanotide, for the treatment of genetic obesity [21]. On the other hand, in fasting conditions, ghrelin and peptide YY (PYY)—the hunger hormones secreted from the stomach and intestine, respectively—activate the AgRP/NPY neurons in the ARC nucleus, which project not only to the PVN but also to the LHA [7,22] (Figure 1). Ghrelin is secreted from the stomach mainly during starvation. The hypothalamus is the brain region that contains the highest density of ghrelin receptors, and some authors showed that ghrelin administration activates neurons in different areas of the hypothalamus, such as the ARC, VMH, and PVN [23] (Figure 1).

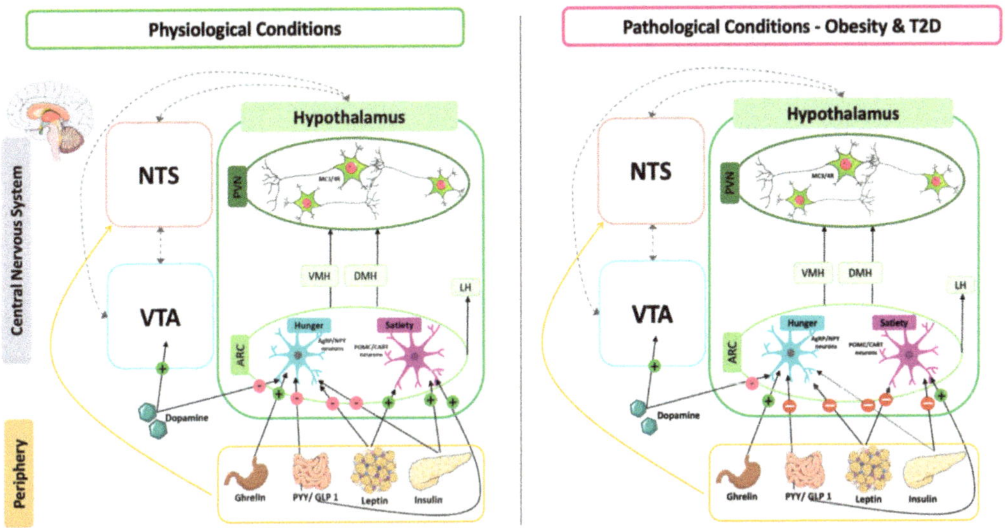

Figure 1. Schematic representation of the brain's satiety network. The left panel shows the neurochemistry and brain network involved in the physiological regulation of feeding behaviour and energy homeostasis and the right panel shows the same network and neurochemistry in pathological conditions, such as obesity and type 2 diabetes. Peripheral signals, such as ghrelin, PYY, GLP1, leptin, and insulin, act in certain regions of the CNS, namely the NTS, hypothalamus, and VTA. Within the hypothalamus, specifically in the ARC nucleus, the satiety-related POMC/CART neurons are activated by insulin, leptin, and GLP 1, and the hunger-related AgRP/NPY neurons are inhibited by PYY, leptin, and dopamine, and activated by ghrelin. Neuronal activity modulation of the ARC nucleus by these peripheral signals will promote alterations in other nuclei of the hypothalamus. In pathological conditions, such as obesity and type 2 diabetes, many of the peripheral signals that modulate ARC nucleus neuronal activity are impaired, with the main relevance for the blocking of insulin, leptin, and ghrelin. AgRP/NPY—neuropeptide Y-agouti-related peptide expressing neurons; ARC—arcuate nucleus; DA—dopamine; DMH—dorsal medial hypothalamus; GLP-1—glucagon-like peptide 1; LH—lateral hypothalamus; NTS—nucleus tractus solitarius; POMC/CART—pro-opiomelanocortin and cocaine- and amphetamine-regulated transcript neurons; PYY—peptide YY; VMH—ventral medial hypothalamus; VTA—ventral tegmental area.

NPY is released by the AgRP/NPY neurons to trigger the increase in food intake and reduce sympathetic activity and BAT thermogenesis, therefore modulating energy expenditure via the activating NPY type 1 receptor at the PVN, which is important in controlling the energy expenditure [24]. Additionally, AgRP can act as an inverse agonist of MC3/4 receptors preventing the anorexigenic effects of α-MSH, which may lead to a decrease in the sympathetic nervous system of the BAT and decreasing thermogenesis [7]. The AgRP/NPY neurons also have an important role in controlling POMC/CART neuronal activity since they can inhibit it via the inhibitory γ-aminobutyric acid (GABA) action. It is also important to note that both POMC/CART and AgRP/NPY neurons at the ARC nucleus receive information from glutamatergic neurons from other hypothalamic nuclei, such as the VMH and the PVN. In contrast, the PVN receives inhibitory innervation from the LHA, which triggers the balance of feeding and regulate energy expenditure by decreasing food intake [25]. Another important brain nucleus regulating food intake, and whose information is integrated into the hypothalamus is the NTS. The NTS, in the caudal brainstem, is the first region in the brain that receives information from the alimentary tract, which is important in the control of food intake. In the NTS, a variety of nutrient, chemical, gastrointestinal–mechanical, and gut peptide signals are first integrated to control energy intake and food ingestion. The NTS is composed of different types of neuronal populations, including the ones containing elements of melanocortinergic and leptinergic signalling, crucial mediators of feeding behaviour regulation. Moreover, the ventral tegmental area (VTA) and the nucleus accumbens (NAc), two brain nuclei, are very important in controlling "hedonic" hunger, and receive projections directly from hypothalamic regions as well as from the LHA. All these brain regions constitute the mesolimbic reward system [26,27]. A lot of attention has been given recently to this mesolimbic reward system, due to its important role in the control of hedonic behaviour. The term hedonic eating refers to the intake of food driven by the reward experienced (rather than metabolic need), which is particularly relevant for cheap, highly palatable, energy-dense foods [28]. Recent studies showed that, in mice, when the inhibitory GABAergic neurons are activated in the LHA, neurons project to the VTA, and animals increase their food intake mainly due to the motivated behaviour to receive a reward [27,29]. Moreover, the activation of GABAergic neurons that project from the LHA to the VTA leads to compulsive sucrose drinking in animals, showing the importance of other circuits other than the hypothalamus in the control of food behaviour [7,27,29].

3. Deregulation of Satiety Pathways in Type 2 Diabetes and Obesity

Glucose is the primary energy source used by humans; it is crucial in maintaining the body's functions. The major hallmark of T2D is hyperglycaemia, which results from defects in insulin production and secretion [4,30]. This state is caused by a wavering of the regulatory circuits that maintain glucose levels within the normal range. One of the major factors that can influence the normal levels of glucose in the organism is the consumption of calorie-rich and high-fat (HF) diets. The increase in caloric intake leads to excessive adipose tissue accumulation, triggering the imbalance between what is consumed and what is spent by the organism. Several circuits and organs are required to maintain glucose homeostasis, with the brain and, particularly, the hypothalamus (the nutrient/hormone-sensing nucleus) playing central roles. In fact, the hypothalamus is not only involved in the physiological regulation of glucose homeostasis, but its deregulation (or at least the deregulation of some circuits/nuclei) contributes to the development of obesity and T2D. For example, it was reported that the ingestion of a HF diet during few days promoted an increase in the amount of saturated fatty acids (FAs) crossing the blood–brain barrier, triggering an inflammatory response in the hypothalamic neuronal population [31]. This phenomenon activates microglia and endoplasmic reticulum (ER) stress culminating in the development of central insulin and leptin resistance [32,33]. Obese individuals and some T2D patients are hyperleptinemic, due to the increased adipose tissue mass. This hyperleptinemic state results in a decrease in the ability of leptin to suppress appetite or increase the body's energy use, causing a constant increase in body weight. The inability of the body to respond to leptin is called leptin resistance [34]. Additionally, in the early stages, they are hyperinsulinemic due to the effort of maintaining normoglycemia in a state of insulin resistance [35]. In the hypothalamus, leptin and insulin resistance can result from the overactivation of their signalling cascades. In the case of leptin resistance, increased levels of leptin could lead to chronic activation of the signal transducer and the activator of transcription-3/suppressor of cytokine signalling 3 (STAT3/SOCS3), a downstream pathway activated by leptin [36]. This will, in turn, inhibit STAT3 signalling via negative feedback, resulting in leptin resistance and insulin resistance [37]. Thus, obesity and T2D are associated with selective insulin and leptin resistance in the hypothalamus, leading to hyperphagic behaviours, alterations in glucose metabolism, and weight gain [38]. In agreement, studies performed on mice with leptin production deficiency, Lep$^{ob/ob}$ (mutations in the gene responsible for the production of leptin) and Lep$^{db/db}$ (leptin-resistance mice due to mutations in leptin receptors) [39] showed hyperphagic behaviours with impaired thermogenesis, which is associated with increased expressions of AgRP and NPY and a decreased expression of α-MSH in POMC [40]. Moreover, several studies have been performed to understand the role of brain insulin in maintaining glucose homeostasis and energy supply to the body. Several studies support that insulin might regulate NPY expression since acute insulin administration in the brain was able to reduce NPY levels in the ARC [41]. Moreover, NPY levels in the hypothalamus were shown to be increased in a rodent model of dysmetabolism, in diabetic rats injected with streptozotocin (STZ) [42]. Apart from controlling the sympathetic outflow from the PVN to the BAT and promoting an increase in thermogenesis, NPY regulates the parasympathetic outflow to the pancreas, stimulating insulin secretion [43]. These findings support the idea that insulin can control NPY levels and functions and vice-versa. Moreover, while the total lack of brain insulin receptors (IRs) leads to T2D and obese phenotypes, mice with the deletion of IRs only in the AgRP and POMC neurons do not exhibit alterations in food intake and energy homeostasis [40]. These findings clearly indicate that there are other neuronal populations apart from AgRP and POMC neurons that could be involved in the control of the central regulation of feeding by insulin, or that AgRP and POMC are not the primary integrators of insulin information-regulating feeding in the brain [41]. Nevertheless, the consumption of hypercaloric diets leading to T2D and obesity is not only associated with the impairment of leptin and insulin signalling in the hypothalamus. There is also some evidence that hypercaloric diets impair the action of ghrelin. During food deprivation, ghrelin levels increase; this is a critical signal to induce hunger during fasting. Surprisingly, and in contrast to what would be expected for an orexigenic hormone, obesity is associated, in humans and rodents, with reduced secretion and ghrelin plasma levels (for a review see [44]). In addition, in obese patients, ghrelin levels do not decrease after meals; this is consistent with the state of ghrelin resistance [44]. Several mechanisms have been postulated to justify the existence of leptin resistance in obesity, including the lower NPY/AgRP responsiveness to plasma ghrelin and the suppression of the neuroendocrine ghrelin axis [45]. This limited action of ghrelin in the hypothalamus observed in HF diet-fed animals promotes a decrease in food intake, which may be an adaptative response to prevent an increase in food intake in individuals with dysmetabolism. Nonetheless, in the PVN, ghrelin action is unaltered, which may indicate that the increase in adiposity is independent of food intake [45,46]. Although the deregulation of the satiety pathways presumes a massive impact on the development of obesity and T2D, it seems that it is not the only intervenient in the control of food behaviour and energy homeostasis, with the reward/reinforcement circuits playing a crucial role in these diseases. Recent studies demonstrated that gut hormones, such as ghrelin, PYY, and GLP-1, can modulate the response of the brain reward regions to nutrient stimuli [47].

We can conclude that homeostatic and reward circuits act together to balance eating between conditions of fasting or lack of food and conditions of overnutrition and that the disruption of these neurocircuits contributes to increased food intake, culminating in dysmetabolic states. Moreover, different types and compositions of hypercaloric diets might differentially impact these neuronal circuits regulating food behaviours. For example, increased levels of ceramides (types of saturated FAs) in the hypothalamus impair the hypothalamic control of food intake and energy expenditure [48]. Furthermore, in vitro studies performed with the hypothalamic neuronal cell line mHypoE-44 showed that prolonged exposure to palmitate attenuates insulin signalling in this hypothalamic neuronal cell line and promotes ER stress in neuronal cells, triggering lipid toxicity [49]. Additionally, in vivo studies showed that the ingestion of HF diets by animals (until there was a 10% increase in their body weights, which typically took 5–7 weeks) [50], led to an increase in hypothalamic cholesterol levels when compared to mice that were submitted to low-fat diets, with consequent increases in food intake and body weight [48]. In another study performed in Zucker rats, an animal model of genetic obesity caused by a mutation in the gene encoding the receptor of leptin showed a link between hypothalamic ER stress caused by the increase in ceramides and the role of the nuclei in energy balance. These authors observed that hypothalamic lipid toxicity leads to a decrease in BAT sympathetic tonus and that the genetic modulation of the ceramide-induced ER pathway in the VMH increases the sympathetic nervous system-mediated BAT thermogenesis, as well as insulin signalling, promoting an overall improvement in the metabolism of the Zucker rats [48,51]. Nevertheless, when talking about the impact of hypercaloric diets on food behaviour, especially in humans, one cannot forget that hypercaloric diets include high percentages of sugars in their composition. In fact, research shows that sugar intake differentially affects the anorexigenic/orexigenic pathways, with sucrose consumption in mice leading to a temporary decrease in orexigenic peptides followed by activation of the orexigenic pathway, potentiating caloric consumption [52]. Moreover, besides the percentage of sugar in the diet, the types of sugars present in the diet may differently impact food behaviour.

4. Impact of Sugar Consumption on Food Behaviour

Sugars are carbohydrates that include fructose and glucose (monosaccharides), and lactose and sucrose (disaccharides), playing different roles in the organism. Sugars can be categorised as (1) intrinsic/natural and (2) extrinsic/added, depending on if they are present in the food without processing, or if they are added. Sucrose, fructose, glucose, starch hydrolysates, and other isolated sugar preparations added during food preparation and manufacturing are included in the added sugars category [53]. It seems consensual that added sugars have a noxious role in the development of metabolic diseases and that sugars that are intrinsically present in food seem to have more harmless impacts on dysmetabolic conditions [54,55]. For example, in a study performed by Monteiro-Alfredo [55], it was shown, in Goto-Kakizaki rats, that the ad libitum ingestion of sugary solutions for 4 weeks impaired energy balance regulation, leading to higher caloric intake, weight gain, fasting hyperglycaemia, insulin intolerance, and impaired oxidative stress/glycation markers than the ad libitum intake of fruit juices, demonstrating the different impacts of added vs intrinsically present sugars in the metabolism.

Importantly, we cannot oversimplify the impact of the different added sugars as it seems that they differently affect satiety pathways. For example, it was shown that the intracerebroventricular administration of glucose and fructose have contrary effects on food intake, with glucose suppressing food intake via the inactivation of hypothalamic AMP-kinase causing the activation of malonyl–CoA signalling system and fructose having inverse effects and, thereby, increasing food intake [56]. These results agree with the data found in a more recent study performed on rats, where the effects of 24 h of free access to different sugars, e.g., sucrose, glucose, fructose, or high-fructose corn syrup on hypothalamic appetite regulation were accessed. The authors observed that glucose consumption resulted in the upregulation of seven satiety-related hypothalamic peptides, including cholecystokinin (CCK), whereas fructose decreased CCK, suggesting that glucose might have a greater impact in promoting satiety when compared to fructose [57]. Interestingly, high fructose corn syrup, a sweetener commonly used to enhance the flavour of foods and beverages, as well as sucrose, had no effect on hypothalamic CCK [57], suggesting that the deregulation of other neural mediators might be involved in the deregulation of hypothalamic pathways by these sugars. Another thing that should be taken into consideration is the fact that these studies were performed in response to acute administrated sugars and that the probability of the long-term intake of sugars might have different effects on hypothalamic satiety pathways. In a study dedicated to evaluating the effects of sucrose, glucose, and fructose in peripheral and central signals, the authors tested their effects after 24 h, 1 week, and 2 weeks of administration in rats and found that long-term exposure to the different sugars differently impacted satiety pathways [58]. Moreover, they found that a 2-week intake of sugar solutions resulted in the downregulation of hypothalamic NPY mRNA, in which a sucrose or fructose solution leads to the upregulation of hypothalamic

CB1 mRNA, and that glucose or fructose downregulated hypothalamic POMC mRNA [58]. In accordance with these results and with the role of endocannabinoids in the regulation of sugar intake, the ingestion of fructose for 1 week was found to affect enzymes involved in the synthesis and degradation of hypothalamic endocannabinoids [59]. Nevertheless, these results might not be so easily translatable to humans. Some authors have found that sugar intake, fructose and glucose, modified serum PYY without changing plasma leptin and ghrelin levels [60], which contrasts with the data found in rats [58]. Moreover, they found that—by using magnetic resonance imaging—glucose, but not fructose, was able to quickly (within 15 min) mediate satiety by reducing brain activity in the hypothalamus [60]. Of interest, they also found that glucose intake induced an increase in functional connectivity between the hypothalamus and striatum, suggesting that glucose improves the communication between appetite control centres.

Apart from impacting hypothalamic satiety pathways, sugar also impacts reward systems due to its additive, palatable, and rewarding characteristics, which may lead to compulsive eating [30,61]. As described in Section 2, hypothalamic neurocircuits project to the mesolimbic pathway, which is composed of the VTA and the NAc, called the reward system, and is important in the control of hedonic hunger [7,16]. Dopamine (DA) is an important neurotransmitter that is involved in functions, such as cognition, emotive behaviour, reward, and memory, also playing a critical role in the control of feeding behaviour and food intake [62]. It is a master regulator of food intake via the mesolimbic neurocircuit by modulating the motivational processes associated with appetite, through its projections from the VTA into the NAc and from the NAc to the hypothalamus [62]. In humans, the ingestion of palatable food promotes the release of DA in the dorsal striatum in proportion to the self-reported level of pleasure derived from eating food [63]. Moreover, upon first exposure to a food reward, DA neurons in VTA increased their firing, resulting in an increase in DA release in NAc [64]. However, the involvement of DA in the reward is more complex than the mere encoding of the hedonic value. Some reports have shown that metabolic mediators from the periphery, such as leptin, insulin, and ghrelin interact with DA in the brain [22]. The increased consumption of foods enriched in sugars can impair the homeostatic mechanisms that control eating behaviour, as in the cases of the dopaminergic pathways. This may lead to overweight, T2D, and obesity states. Previous studies performed on animals and humans showed that glucose as well as sucrose [65] modulate DA activity in the VTA and substantia nigra. More recently, it was shown that post-ingestive sucrose, but not sucralose—an artificial sweetener and sugar substitute—can sustain operant food-seeking behaviour, which is an effect be mediated the activation of a subpopulation of VTA dopamine neurons via the vagus nerve [66]. Sucrose is broken down into fructose and glucose molecules and, therefore, fructose may possess reinforcing properties activating the reward system, such as sucrose. In fact, it has been shown that fructose activates reward-related regions within the mesocorticolimbic DA system, as seen by c-Fos induction in the dorsal striatum and amygdala in rats, increases the BOLD signal in the dorsal striatum, pre-frontal cortex, and orbitofrontal cortex of pigs, and increases dopamine levels in the VTA (for a review, see [67]). Moreover, it was shown that fructose-mediated cortical disinhibition increases impulsivity toward food rewards, potentiating overfeeding [67]. Overall, we can conclude that different sugars differently regulate hunger and satiety but also food-seeking and reward pathways.

Furthermore, the effects of sugars on the modulation of dopamine pathways in the mesolimbic system might not be direct and could involve the release of hormones in the periphery and the interaction with the dopaminergic pathways [68]. Insulin, ghrelin, leptin, and GLP-1 interact with DA neurons in the midbrain [68–71]. Leptin and insulin inhibit DA neurons while ghrelin triggers its activation. Insulin is known to promote the desire for fat and sugars, reducing hedonic feeding. Moreover, upon injections of leptin in the VTA, food intake is reduced, and the ablation of leptin receptors in this region increases the reward of palatable meals, which include sugars. In the presence of dysmetabolism states, the modulation of dopaminergic pathways with DA agonists triggers weight loss in obese animals through the activation of dopamine type 1 (D1R) and type 2 receptors (D2R), although D2R is more associated with food seeking, motivation, and satiety inhibitory control [72]. Additionally, hyperphagia in obese mice is attenuated with DA administration and reward.

5. Conclusions

In conclusion, we provide evidence that not all sugars are equally deleterious in affecting the control of food behaviours, as they have different impacts on the deregulation of satiety and reward pathways leading to obesity and T2D. Knowing that food behaviours involve complex and multifaceted interplays of mechanisms, driven not only by hunger/satiety but also by cravings and hedonic memories, more attention and research should be performed to study the impacts of the different sugars in these pathways, which are particularly important in states of dysmetabolism, such as obesity and T2D.

Author Contributions: Conceptualization, A.M.C. and S.V.C.; writing—review and editing, A.M.C. and S.V.C. All authors have read and agreed to the published version of the manuscript.

Funding: This study was supported by the Portuguese Foundation for Science with a research grant EXPL/MED-NEU/0733/2021.

Institutional Review Board Statement: Not applicable.

Informed Consent Statement: Not applicable.

Data Availability Statement: The data presented in this study are available on request from the corresponding author.

Conflicts of Interest: The authors declare no conflict of interest.

References

1. Egger, G.; Dixon, J. Beyond obesity and lifestyle: A review of 21st century chronic disease determinants. *Biomed. Res. Int.* **2014**, *2014*, 731685. [CrossRef] [PubMed]
2. Golay, A.; Ybarra, J. Link between obesity and type 2 diabetes. *Best Pract. Res. Clin. Endocrinol. Metab.* **2005**, *19*, 649–663. [CrossRef] [PubMed]
3. International Diabetes Federation. *IDF Diabetes*; International Diabetes Federation: Brussels, Belgium, 2019.
4. DeFronzo, R.A. Pathogenesis of type 2 diabetes mellitus. *Med. Clin.* **2004**, *88*, 787–835. [CrossRef] [PubMed]
5. ADA. American Diabetes Association. 2021. Available online: https://www.diabetes.org/diabetes (accessed on 19 November 2022).
6. Wysham, C.; Shubrook, J. Beta-cell failure in type 2 diabetes: Mechanisms, markers, and clinical implications. *Postgrad. Med.* **2020**, *132*, 676–686. [CrossRef] [PubMed]
7. Timper, K.; Brüning, J.C. Hypothalamic circuits regulating appetite and energy homeostasis: Pathways to obesity. *DMM Dis. Model. Mech.* **2017**, *10*, 679–689. [CrossRef] [PubMed]
8. Billes, S.K.; Simonds, S.E.; Cowley, M.A. Leptin reduces food intake via a dopamine D2 receptor-dependent mechanism. *Mol. Metab.* **2012**, *1*, 86–93. [CrossRef]
9. Khodai, T.; Luckman, S.M. Ventromedial Nucleus of the Hypothalamus Neurons under the Magnifying Glass. *Endocrinology* **2021**, *162*, bqab141. [CrossRef]
10. Hetherington, A.W.; Ranson, S.W. The relation of various hypothalamic lesions to adiposity in the rat. *J. Comp. Neurol.* **1942**, *76*, 475–499. [CrossRef]
11. Delgado, J.M.; Anand, B.K. Increase of food intake induced by electrical stimulation of the lateral hypothalamus. *Am. J. Physiol.* **1953**, *172*, 162–168. [CrossRef]
12. Al-Dossary, A.F.; Al-Majed, A.; Hossain, M.E.; Rahman, M.K.; Jennings, S.; Bargawi, R. The Need to Feed: Homeostatic and Hedonic Control of Eating. In Proceedings of the 17th Middle East Oil & Gas Show and Conference 2011 (MEOS 2011), Manama, Bahrain, 25–28 September 2011; Volume 3, pp. 1660–1672.
13. Anand, B.K.; Brobeck, J.R. Localization of a 'Feeding Center' in the Hypothalamus of the Rat. *Proc. Soc. Exp. Biol. Med.* **1951**, *77*, 323–325. [CrossRef]
14. Stuber, G.D.; Wise, R.A. Lateral hypothalamic circuits for feeding and reward. *Nat. Neurosci.* **2016**, *19*, 198–205. [CrossRef]
15. Ono, T.; Nakamura, K.; Nishijo, H.; Fukuda, M. Hypothalamic neuron involvement in integration of reward, aversion, and cue signals. *J. Neurophysiol.* **1986**, *56*, 63–79. [CrossRef]
16. Valassi, E.; Scacchi, M.; Cavagnini, F. Neuroendocrine control of food intake. *Nutr. Metab. Cardiovasc. Dis.* **2008**, *18*, 158–168. [CrossRef]
17. Hruby, V.J.; Cone, R.D. Role of melanocortinergic neurons in feeding and the agouti obesity syndrome. *Nature* **1997**, *385*, 165–168.

18. Marie, L.S.; Miura, G.I.; Marsh, D.J.; Yagaloff, K.; Palmiter, R.D. A metabolic defect promotes obesity in mice lacking melanocortin-4 receptors. *Proc. Natl. Acad. Sci. USA* **2000**, *97*, 12339–12344. [CrossRef]
19. Voss-Andreae, A.; Murphy, J.G.; Ellacott, K.L.J.; Stuart, R.C.; Nillni, E.A.; Cone, R.D.; Fan, W. Role of the central melanocortin circuitry in adaptive thermogenesis of brown adipose tissue. *Endocrinology* **2007**, *148*, 1550–1560. [CrossRef]
20. Vaisse, C.; Clement, K.; Guy-Grand, B.; Froguel, P. A frameshift mutation in human MC4R is associated with a dominant form of obesity. *Nat. Genet.* **1998**, *20*, 113–114. [CrossRef]
21. Markham, A. Setmelanotide: First Approval. *Drugs* **2021**, *81*, 397–403. [CrossRef]
22. Ahima, R.S.; Antwi, D.A. Brain Regulation of Appetite and Satiety. *Endocrinol. Metab. Clin. North Am.* **2008**, *37*, 811–823. [CrossRef]
23. Tong, J.; D'Alessio, D. Ghrelin and hypothalamic development: Too little and too much of a good thing. *J. Clin. Investig.* **2015**, *125*, 490–492. [CrossRef]
24. Huang, Y.; Lin, X.; Lin, S. Neuropeptide Y and Metabolism Syndrome: An Update on Perspectives of Clinical Therapeutic Intervention Strategies. *Front. Cell Dev. Biol.* **2021**, *9*, 695623. [CrossRef] [PubMed]
25. Waterson, M.J.; Horvath, T.L. Neuronal Regulation of Energy Homeostasis: Beyond the Hypothalamus and Feeding. *Cell Metab.* **2015**, *22*, 962–970. [CrossRef] [PubMed]
26. Schwartz, G.J. Integrative capacity of the caudal brainstem in the control of food intake. *Philos. Trans. R. Soc. B Biol. Sci.* **2006**, *361*, 1275–1280. [CrossRef] [PubMed]
27. Tyree, S.M.; de Lecea, L. Lateral hypothalamic control of the ventral tegmental area: Reward evaluation and the driving of motivated behavior. *Front. Syst. Neurosci.* **2017**, *11*, 50. [CrossRef] [PubMed]
28. Lowe, M.R.; Butryn, M.L. Hedonic hunger: A new dimension of appetite? *Physiol. Behav.* **2007**, *91*, 432–439. [CrossRef]
29. Castro, D.C.; Cole, S.L.; Berridge, K.C. Lateral hypothalamus, nucleus accumbens, and ventral pallidum roles in eating and hunger: Interactions between homeostatic and reward circuitry. *Front. Syst. Neurosci.* **2015**, *9*, 90. [CrossRef]
30. Capucho, A.; Chegão, A.; Martins, F.; Miranda, H.V.; Conde, S. Dysmetabolism and Neurodegeneration: Trick or Treat? *Nutrients* **2022**, *14*, 1425. [CrossRef]
31. Ruth, M. Obesity is associated with hypothalamic injury in rodents and humans. *Yearb. Endocrinol.* **2012**, *2012*, 119–120. [CrossRef]
32. Schneeberger, M.; Dietrich, M.O.; Sebastián, D.; Imbernón, M.; Castaño, C.; Garcia, A.; Esteban, Y.; Gonzalez-Franquesa, A.; Rodríguez, I.C.; Bortolozzi, A.; et al. Mitofusin 2 in POMC neurons connects ER stress with leptin resistance and energy imbalance. *Cell* **2013**, *155*, 172–187. [CrossRef]
33. Zhang, X.; Zhang, G.; Zhang, H.; Karin, M.; Bai, H.; Cai, D. Hypothalamic IKKβ/NF-kB and ER stress Link Overnutrition. *Cell* **2009**, *135*, 61–73. [CrossRef]
34. Farr, O.M.; Gavirieli, A. What have we learned about leptin and obesity. *Physiol. Behav.* **2017**, *176*, 139–148.
35. Ambwani, R.K.S.; Misra, A.K. Evaluation of Leptin as a Marker of Insulin Resistance in Type 2 Diabetes Mellitus. *Int. J. Appl. Basic Med. Res.* **2017**, *2019*, 193–195.
36. Vaisse, C.; Halaas, J.L.; Horvath, C.M.; Darnell, J.E.; Stoffel, M.; Friedman, J.M. Leptin activation of Stat3 in the hypothalamus of wild–type and ob/ob mice but not db/db mice. *Nat. Genet.* **1996**, *14*, 95–97. [CrossRef]
37. Ernst, M.B.; Wunderlich, C.M.; Hess, S.; Paehler, M.; Mesaros, A.; Koralov, S.; Kleinridders, A.; Husch, A.; Münzberg, H.; Hampel, B.; et al. Enhanced Stat3 activation in POMC neurons provokes negative feedback inhibition of leptin and insulin signaling in obesity. *J. Neurosci.* **2009**, *29*, 11582–11593. [CrossRef]
38. Könner, A.C.; Brüning, J.C. Selective insulin and leptin resistance in metabolic disorders. *Cell Metab.* **2012**, *16*, 144–152. [CrossRef]
39. Suriano, F.; Vieira-Silva, S.; Falony, G.; Roumain, M.; Paquot, A.; Pelicaen, R.; Régnier, M.; Delzenne, N.M.; Raes, J.; Muccioli, G.G.; et al. Novel insights into the genetically obese (ob/ob) and diabetic (db/db) mice: Two sides of the same coin. *Microbiome* **2021**, *9*, 147. [CrossRef]
40. Ahima, R.S.; Saper, C.B.; Flier, J.S.; Elmquist, J.K. Leptin regulation of neuroendocrine systems. *Front. Neuroendocrinol.* **2000**, *21*, 263–307. [CrossRef]
41. Loh, K.; Zhang, L.; Brandon, A.; Wang, Q.; Begg, D.; Qi, Y.; Fu, M.; Kulkarni, R.; Teo, J.; Baldock, P.; et al. Insulin controls food intake and energy balance via NPY neurons. *Mol. Metab.* **2017**, *6*, 574–584. [CrossRef]
42. Gelling, R.W.; Morton, G.J.; Morrison, C.; Niswender, K.D.; Myers, M.G.; Rhodes, C.J.; Schwartz, M.W. Insulin action in the brain contributes to glucose lowering during insulin treatment of diabetes. *Cell Metab.* **2006**, *3*, 67–73. [CrossRef]
43. Cassaglia, P.A.; Shi, Z.; Brooks, V.L. Insulin increases sympathetic nerve activity in part by suppression of tonic inhibitory neuropeptide y inputs into the paraventricular nucleus in female rats. *Am. J. Physiol. Regul. Integr. Comp. Physiol.* **2016**, *311*, R97–R103. [CrossRef]
44. Cui, H.; López, M.; Rahmouni, K. The cellular and molecular bases of leptin and ghrelin resistance in obesity. *Nat. Rev. Endocrinol.* **2017**, *13*, 338–351. [CrossRef] [PubMed]
45. Briggs, D.I.; Enriori, P.J.; Lemus, M.B.; Cowley, M.; Andrews, Z.B. Diet-induced obesity causes ghrelin resistance in arcuate NPY/AgRP neurons. *Endocrinology* **2010**, *151*, 4745–4755. [CrossRef] [PubMed]
46. Shrestha, Y.B.; Wickwire, K.; Giraudo, S. Effect of reducing hypothalamic ghrelin receptor gene expression on energy balance. *Peptides* **2009**, *30*, 1336–1341. [CrossRef] [PubMed]
47. Decarie-Spain, L.; Kanoski, S. Ghrelin and glucagon-like peptide-1: A gut-brain axis battle for food reward. *Nutrients* **2021**, *13*, 977. [CrossRef] [PubMed]

48. González-Garciá, I.; Fernø, J.; Diéguez, C.; Nogueiras, R.; López, M. Hypothalamic Lipids: Key Regulators of Whole Body Energy Balance. *Neuroendocrinology* **2017**, *104*, 398–411. [CrossRef]
49. Mayer, C.M.; Belsham, D.D. Palmitate attenuates insulin signaling and induces endoplasmic reticulum stress and apoptosis in hypothalamic neurons: Rescue of resistance and apoptosis through adenosine 5′ monophosphate-activated protein kinase activation. *Endocrinology* **2010**, *151*, 576–585. [CrossRef]
50. Posey, K.A.; Clegg, D.J.; Printz, R.L.; Byun, J.; Morton, G.J.; Vivekanandan-Giri, A.; Pennathur, S.; Baskin, D.G.; Heinecke, J.W. Woods, S.C.; et al. Hypothalamic proinflammatory lipid accumulation, inflammation, and insulin resistance in rats fed a high-fat diet. *Am. J. Physiol. Endocrinol. Metab.* **2009**, *296*, E1003–E1012. [CrossRef]
51. Contreras, C.; García, I.G.; Martinez-Sanchez, N.; Seoane-Collazo, P.; Jacas, J.; Morgan, D.A.; Serra, D.; Gallego, R.; Gonzalez F.; Casals, N.; et al. Central ceramide-induced hypothalamic lipotoxicity and ER stress regulate energy balance. *Cell Rep* **2014**, *9*, 366–377. [CrossRef]
52. Gaysinskaya, V.; Karatayev, O.; Shuluk, J.; Leibowitz, S. Hyperphagia induced by sucrose: Relation to circulating and CSF glucose and corticosterone and orexigenic peptides in the arcuate nucleus. *Pharmacol. Biochem. Behav.* **2011**, *97*, 521–530. [CrossRef]
53. European Food Safety Authority (EFSA). Scientific Opinion on establishing Food-Based Dietary Guidelines. *EFSA J.* **2016**, *8*, 1460
54. Martins, F.O.; Conde, S.V. Impact of Diet Composition on Insulin Resistance. *Nutrients* **2022**, *14*, 3716. [CrossRef]
55. Monteiro-Alfredo, T.; Caramelo, B.; Arbeláez, D.; Amaro, A.; Barra, C.; Silva, D.; Oliveira, S.; Seiça, R.; Matafome, P. Distinct impact of natural sugars from fruit juices and added sugars on caloric intake, body weight, glycaemia, oxidative stress and glycation in diabetic rats. *Nutrients* **2021**, *13*, 2956. [CrossRef]
56. Seung, H.C.; Wolfgang, M.; Tokutake, Y.; Chohnan, S.; Lane, M.D. Differential effects of central fructose and glucose on hypothalamic malonyl-CoA and food intake. *Proc. Natl. Acad. Sci. USA* **2008**, *105*, 16871–16875.
57. Colley, D.L.; Castonguay, T.W. Effects of sugar solutions on hypothalamic appetite regulation. *Physiol. Behav.* **2015**, *139*, 202–209 [CrossRef]
58. Lindqvist, A.; Baelemans, A.; Erlanson-Albertsson, C. Effects of sucrose, glucose and fructose on peripheral and central appetite signals. *Regul. Pept.* **2008**, *150*, 26–32. [CrossRef]
59. Erlanson-Albertsson, C.; Lindqvist, A. Fructose affects enzymes involved in the synthesis and degradation of hypothalamic endocannabinoids. *Regul. Pept.* **2010**, *161*, 87–91. [CrossRef]
60. Page, K.A.; Chan, O.; Arora, J.; Belfort-Deaguiar, R.; Dzuira, J.; Roehmholdt, B.; Cline, G.W.; Naik, S.; Sinha, R.; Constable, R.T.; et al. Effects of Fructose vs Glucose on Regional Cerebral Blood Flow in Brain Regions Involved with Appetite and Reward Pathways. *JAMA* **2013**, *39*, 63–70. [CrossRef]
61. Freeman, C.; Zehra, A.; Ramirex, V.; Wiers, C.; Volkow, N.; Wang, G.-J. Impact of Sugar on the Body. *Front. Biosci.* **2018**, *23*, 2255–2266.
62. Volkow, N.D.; Wang, G.-J.; Baler, R.D. Reward, dopamine and the control of food intake: Implications for obesity. *Trends Cogn. Sci.* **2012**, *15*, 37–46. [CrossRef]
63. Small, D.M.; Jones-Gotman, M.; Dagher, A. Feeding-induced dopamine release in dorsal striatum correlates with meal pleasantness ratings in healthy human volunteers. *Neuroimage* **2003**, *19*, 1709–1715. [CrossRef]
64. Range, K.D.M.; Moser, Y.A. Gustatory Reward and the Nucleus Accumbens. *Physiol. Behav.* **2012**, *23*, 531–535.
65. Eiler, W.J.; Dzemidzic, M.; Soeurt, C.M.; Carron, C.R.; Oberlin, B.G.; Considine, R.V.; Harezlak, J.; Kareken, D.A. Family history of alcoholism and the human brain response to oral sucrose. *NeuroImage Clin.* **2018**, *17*, 1036–1046. [CrossRef] [PubMed]
66. Fernandes, A.B.; da Silva, J.A.; Almeida, J.; Cui, G.; Gerfen, C.R.; Costa, R.M.; Oliveira-Maia, A.J. Postingestive Modulation of Food Seeking Depends on Vagus-Mediated Dopamine Neuron Activity. *Neuron* **2020**, *106*, 778–788.e6. [CrossRef] [PubMed]
67. Payant, M.A.; Chee, M.J. Neural mechanisms underlying the role of fructose in overfeeding. *Neurosci. Biobehav. Rev.* **2021**, *128*, 346–357. [CrossRef]
68. Wang, G.J.; Volkow, N.D.; Thanos, P.K.; Fowler, J.S. Imaging of brain dopamine pathways: Implications for understanding obesity. *J. Addict. Med.* **2009**, *3*, 8–18. [CrossRef]
69. Adam, T.C.; Epel, E.S. Stress, eating and the reward system. *Physiol. Behav.* **2007**, *91*, 449–458. [CrossRef]
70. Palmiter, R.D. Is dopamine a physiologically relevant mediator of feeding behavior? *Trends Neurosci.* **2007**, *30*, 375–381. [CrossRef]
71. Abizaid, A.; Liu, Z.-W.; Andrews, Z.B.; Shanabrough, M.; Borok, E.; Elsworth, J.D.; Roth, R.H.; Sleeman, M.W.; Picciotto, M.; Tschöp, M.H.; et al. Ghrelin modulates the activity and synaptic input organization of midbrain dopamine neurons while promoting appetite. *J. Clin. Investig.* **2006**, *116*, 3229–3239. [CrossRef]
72. Missale, C.; Nash, S.R.; Robinson, S.W.; Jaber, M.; Caron, M.G. Dopamine receptors: From structure to function. *Physiol. Rev.* **1998**, *78*, 189–225. [CrossRef]

diabetology

MDPI

Opinion

Dietary Sugars during Critical Phases of Development and Long-Term Risk of Non-Communicable Diseases

Marcos Divino Ferreira-Junior, Keilah Valéria Naves Cavalcante, Ariel Penha Carvalho da Mota and Rodrigo Mello Gomes *

Laboratory of Endocrine Physiology and Metabolism, Biological Sciences Institute, Federal University of Goiás, Goiania 746900-900, Brazil; marcosdfjunior@gmail.com (M.D.F.-J.); keilah1506@gmail.com (K.V.N.C.); arielmota.ufg@gmail.com (A.P.C.d.M.)
* Correspondence: gomesrm@ufg.br

Abstract: Obesity and the intake of high-sugar diets have dramatically increased in recent decades. However, it is still uncertain how sugar intake during the critical development phase affects the long-term health of children. In this context, the Developmental Origins of Health and Disease (DOHaD) concept established a correlation between early life environment and the development of cardiometabolic diseases in adulthood. This review summarizes the current knowledge about the consequences of sugar intake during the critical development phase for the onset of non-communicable diseases (NCDs). We found evidence that increased sugar intake during pregnancy contributes to maternal obesity and many cardiometabolic dysfunctions in the offspring. Furthermore, dietary sugar during the suckling period provokes the obese phenotype in adulthood. Finally, high-sugar diet intake during childhood induces metabolic syndrome and depressive-like behavior.

Keywords: DOHaD; pregnancy; lactation; childhood; obesity

Citation: Ferreira-Junior, M.D.; Cavalcante, K.V.N.; Mota, A.P.C.d.; Gomes, R.M. Dietary Sugars during Critical Phases of Development and Long-Term Risk of Non-Communicable Diseases. *Diabetology* **2023**, *4*, 243–250. https://doi.org/10.3390/diabetology4030021

Academic Editor: Peter Clifton

Received: 17 May 2023
Revised: 19 June 2023
Accepted: 21 June 2023
Published: 25 June 2023

1. Introduction

It is evident that obesity is a public health concern around the world. According to the World Health Organization (WHO), worldwide obesity has nearly tripled since 1975, and there are around 2 billion adults who are overweight and 650 million who are obese. In 2016, it is estimated that more that 40 million children under the age of 5 years were overweight or obese. Moreover, between 1975 and 2016, the prevalence of obesity among children and adolescents increased from 4% to 18% [1].

Maternal and childhood obesity is linked to a range of adverse health outcomes later in life, as well as some negative societal outcomes. Recent studies have shown an association between nutritional insults during the initial phases of development and a long-term risk of non-communicable diseases (NCDs), including obesity, diabetes and cardiovascular diseases [2,3]. Thus, the developmental origins of the health and disease hypothesis (DOHaD) proposes a link between the fetal, early infant and puberty phases of life and the long-term development of cardiometabolic disorders [4]. This is why we consider the governmental and private strategies linked to the DOHaD concept one of our political priorities.

The main mechanisms, according to the DOHaD hypothesis, are epigenetic adaptations, such as DNA methylation, histone acetylation and differential small RNAs expression, that occur during critical phases of development in response to environmental factors like nutritional disorders [5].

In general, increased calorie intake and decreased physical activity play a key role in obesity onset and in the most common causes of NCDs [6]. It has been noted that the intake of dietary sugars, mainly sugar-sweetened beverages, increases overall energy intake, leading to a reduced intake of healthy foods containing adequate calories, contributing to body weight gain and increased risk of NCDs [7]. Recently, a study showed that male mice fed a standard diet but drinking sweetened water (60 mg/mL sucrose solution) for sixteen weeks, presented a significant increase in fat mass, leading to increased plasma LDL and insulin, glucose intolerance and hepatic steatosis [8].

Sugar enriched diets contain high levels of monosaccharides (glucose, fructose and galactose) and disaccharides (sucrose, maltose and lactose), which are named as free sugars, and also contain polysaccharides such as starch. In this sense, there is a growing concern about the intake of foods whose caloric content is basically composed by added sugars, mainly sugar-sweetened beverages. The WHO recommends that the intake of free sugars be less than 5% of total energy intake [7]. However, this amount is often exceeded with sugar-sweetened beverages intake. The free sugars are quickly absorbed and contribute significantly to high blood glucose levels, leading to increased insulinemia. In the long term, this condition leads to the development of glucose intolerance and insulin resistance [9]. Furthermore, a high dietary sugar intake contributes to the formation of endogenous advanced glycation end products (AGEs). A high fructose intake is related to AGE accumulation in different tissues, which leads to insulin resistance and dyslipidemia [10]. Studies have reported that perinatal exposure to AGEs during pregnancy and lactation is one of the factors causing metabolic programming, increasing the risk of developing NCDs in adulthood [11].

Unfortunately, it has been reported that the intake of sugary foods is high among children and adolescents [7]. Glucose is the main source of energy to the central nervous system (CNS), and high-sugar diets can provoke an overdrive mode in the CNS. When the CNS is overstimulated by excess sugars, it leads to hyperactivity and mood swings. However, these behavioral changes are not the only short-term consequences. Some evidence suggests that this hyperactivity in the CNS in adolescents is linked to the anxiogenic state in adulthood. Sugar also causes an addictive effect, stimulating neurons of the limbic system, which reinforces further sugar consumption [12].

In this review, we provide updated knowledge about the intake of dietary sugars and their risk for NCDs onset in adults and children. As well as highlighting the importance of recognizing the rapidly growing epidemic of overweight and obesity during critical phases of development, we also explore the adaptive mechanisms of phenotypic changes early in life and the long-term effects supported by the DOHaD concept.

2. Materials and Methods

In this study the relationship between high-sugar diets and DOHaD were assessed by comprehensive literature review. Through advanced search on PubMed, Medline, Scopus and Google Scholar, manuscripts published between January 1990 and December 2022 were assessed and filtered by the following search strategy: "(sugar) AND ((pregnancy) OR (lactation) OR (childhood) OR (puberty) OR (DOHaD) OR (obesity) OR (diabetes) OR (non-communicable diseases))".

The inclusion criteria of the selected manuscripts were studies that showed some kind of relationship between the early intake of a sugary diet and non-communicable diseases in adult life.

3. Dietary Sugars and Pregnancy

Adequate maternal body weight gain during pregnancy is important for ensuring the healthy development of the fetus. Maternal nutrition is one of the main factors that impairs body weight gain of the mother during gestational period. Few studies have specifically evaluated the effects of high-sugar intake on gestational body weight gain. In a cohort study with Danish women, Maslova et al. found that sugar intake during pregnancy was correlated with excessive gestational weight gain (GWG). The authors evaluated the relation between protein/carbohydrate (P/C) ratio and added sugar intake during pregnancy and GWG. This study shows that a high P/C ratio is an important determinant of reduced GWG. On the other hand, high-sugar intake was related to increased GWG, as stated by the authors "added sugar consumption was strongly associated with GWG

(Q5 vs. Q1: 34, 95% CI 28 to 40 g/week)" [13]. In another study, authors have shown that intake of added sugars food, including sweets, snacks, cakes and soft drinks, were strongly associated with body weight gain in pregnant woman, in which women who consumed sweets ≥ 2/day gained an additional 5.4 kg (95% CI 2.1–8.7). The authors also note that reducing the added sugars intake is more important to prevent GWG than reducing the intake of other nutrients, such as protein or saturated fat [14].

Independent of maternal body weight gain or gestational obesity, excessive sugar intake during pregnancy is associated with pregnancy complications, such as gestational diabetes, preeclampsia and premature delivery. The main mechanisms involved in the effects of sugar intake on pregnancy complications are insulin sensitivity and inflammation. In this review, the focus is not exclusively on maternal harm due to greater weight gain during pregnancy, but rather on the consequences for the children of mothers who ingest high-sugar diets. In this sense, Catherine et al. showed that offspring born from mothers fed with 50% fructose were hyperglycemic at birth [15].

The ingestion of high-sugar diets during the gestational period is not only harmful to the pregnant person's or to the fetus' health during uterine life. According to the DOHaD concept, pregnancy is an important stage of ontogenetic plasticity. Arima and Fukuoka have shown that birth weight is inversely associated with the incidence of cardiovascular disease. The authors also presented some studies that point out that maternal malnutrition during pregnancy causes long-term consequences to the offspring, which includes several cardiometabolic dysfunctions [16].

During fetal development, intense neurogenesis occurs. In addition, environmental and nutritional disruptions can interfere with the CNS development, especially in the hypothalamus, which can compromise its function. The hypothalamic-pituitary-adrenal (HPA) axis is dramatically affected during fetal development. Changes in the HPA axis during pregnancy can result in dysfunctions in the release and action of glucocorticoids (corticosterone in rodents and cortisol in humans). It was observed that the offspring from rats fed a standard chow plus 20% (w/v) fructose in drinking water during gestation showed increased circulating corticosterone, and enhanced DNA methylation of 5α-reductase 1 promoter region in the adrenal of the offspring at postnatal day 160 [17]. Rodrigo et al. investigated whether maternal fructose intake (10% w/v in drinking water) by pregnant rats throughout gestation produces changes in the cholesterol metabolism of progeny. The authors observed different responses between the sexes, the male offspring from fructose-fed mothers had higher plasma HDL-cholesterol levels, whereas the female offspring from fructose-fed mothers had lower levels of non-HDL cholesterol. An important result of this study was the increase in the DNA methylation of Liver X-receptor (LXRα) in males from fructose-fed mothers, which decreased in the corresponding group of females. LXRα is an important regulator of cholesterol metabolism [18]. Rodriquez et al. also demonstrated that maternal fructose intake (10% w/v in drinking water) during pregnancy affects maternal and fetal leptin signaling [19]. Vickers et al. similarly demonstrated that offspring from fructose-fed mothers (20% of caloric intake from fructose) had impaired metabolic function, hyperglycemia and hyperleptinemia [20]. Together, these effects may predispose the offspring to obesity and metabolic syndrome later in life, with consequent development of cardiovascular diseases and diabetes.

4. Dietary Sugars and Lactation/Infancy

For rodents, it is perhaps possible that lactation is one of the most critical phases of development. This occurs because the neural differentiation of the circuitry responsible for appetite and energy expenditure begins in the last week of gestation and continues during lactation in rodents [21]. Around the first 14 days after birth, there is an increase in the leptin levels on the blood, which is called a postnatal leptin surge. Therefore, leptin levels during lactation are crucial for the offspring's CNS development [22].

The WHO recommends exclusive breastfeeding until 6 months of life and complementary breastfeeding until the age of 2 years [23]. It has been observed that breastfeeding prevents several diseases such as diabetes, multiple sclerosis, cardiovascular and celiac diseases [24]. Breast milk composition depends on maternal nutrition and there is evidence that breast milk may also be a source of glycotoxins during lactation. Studies have shown that the neonatal intake of breast milk from diabetic mothers was related to overweight and glucose intolerance in the offspring [25].

Our group published a study where it was observed that the offspring of diet-induced obese mothers (DIO, containing sucrose and sweetened condensed milk) throughout the suckling period, presented in the obese phenotype in adulthood. Maternal DIO produces subsequent changes in breast milk composition, increasing carbohydrates and lipids content Furthermore, DIO offspring developed leptin and insulin hypothalamic resistance and peripheral glucose dyshomeostasis, leading to changes in the morphology of the endocrine pancreas, with compensatory pancreatic β-cell hypertrophy [26].

During the first years of life, the central nervous system shows great plasticity and is subject to changes caused by maternal nutritional impairments that can affect the infant's learning. Berger et al. evaluated whether infant cognitive development can be negatively affected maternal fructose consumption. The authors showed that maternal fructose intake during the first postnatal month was negatively correlated with infant cognitive development at two postnatal years [27].

As an effect of the higher consumption of sugars or the formula-feeding of infants, increased levels of glycotoxins such as methylglyoxal (MG) are very harmful to health Francisco et al. [28] evaluated whether maternal MG exposure during lactation programs the progeny to metabolic dysfunction later in life. MG mothers had elevated levels of glucose, triglycerides, cholesterol and fructosamine and low insulin in the breast milk Furthermore, MG offspring had the obese phenotype in adulthood, as well as glucose intolerance and impaired β-cell function. They also showed increased risk of cardiovascular disease [28]. On the other hand, a sugar restricted diet during neonatal period prevented the development of type 1 diabetes in the offspring of non-obese diabetic mice [29]. In addition, infant formulas are rich in sugars and proteins, and their industrial production includes heat treatment, which can increase the amount of the AGEs, such as MG. In humans, Rose et al. [30] described that formula-fed children were more prone to choose unhealthy foods Additionally, Weijs et al. [31] have shown that a high intake of sugar-containing beverages in the first year of life were correlated to a higher risk of developing obesity/overweight in 8-year-old children.

Due to the proximity of the puberty period to the lactation period in animal models, the keywords "infancy" or "childhood" rarely return results. In humans, due to the difficulty of obtaining results through questionnaires, there are few studies of cohorts that evaluate the long-term effects of high sugar intake during the childhood.

5. Dietary Sugars and Puberty

The increased obesity rates among children and adolescents are a great public health problem. In the United States, more than 40% of children and adolescents are overweight or obese. Puberty is an important ontogenetic window due to several morphophysiological changes that occur in this phase. This period is marked by increased of individual freedom, dietary and lifestyle choices, associated with risky behaviors such as smoking and alcohol consumption [32]. In response to concerns about adolescent food choices, the WHO [7] has reduced the recommended intake of free sugars to less than 5% of total energy intake.

According to the Dietary Guidelines for Americans (DGA), adolescent (14 to 18 years old) girls require about 1800 to 2400 calories per day and boys need about 2000 to 3200 calories per day. The foods that make up a healthy dietary pattern include: vegetables, beans, peas, lentils and starchy foods; fruits, especially whole fruit; grains; dairy, including fat-free or low-fat milk, yogurt and cheese, and/or lactose-free versions and fortified soy beverages; protein foods, including lean meats, poultry and eggs; seafood; nuts, seeds and soy products; and oils, including vegetable oils and oils in food, such as seafood and nuts [33]. In addition to physical inactivity, malnutrition among adolescents is the main cause of the increase in the number of obese young people. In this sense, the high intake of free sugars contributes to the increase in NCDs.

Harrell et al. showed that a high-fructose diet intake during adolescence increases neuroinflammation and depressive-like behaviors. Furthermore, the authors also showed that feeding male rats a sugar-rich diet (55% *w*/*w* energy from fructose), provoked elevated TNFα and corticosterone levels [34].

In a recent study, the authors presented the fact that non-natural food intake, of foods containing high fructose levels, was associated with elevated diastolic blood pressure (DBP) in adolescent girls. The authors emphasize that the consumption of natural foods containing fructose, (e.g., fruits) does not impact blood pressure and should continue as part of a healthy diet [35]. On the other hand, Schwimmer et al. observed that adolescent boys with NAFLD had a significant improvement in hepatic steatosis after 8 weeks of eating a diet composed of less than 3% daily calories from free sugar [36]. In the same sense, in another study, the authors showed that the intake of sugars by adolescents in the US is associated with low HDL cholesterol levels, high LDL cholesterol and triglycerides and overweight/obese, known to increase metabolic syndrome risk [37]. In a study that examined the association between added sugar intake and metabolic syndrome, US adolescents (1623), aged 12–19 years, were evaluated. Rodríguez et al. showed that added sugar intake is directly associated with metabolic syndrome among non-Hispanic white, non-Hispanic black and Mexican-American US adolescents, independent of total energy intake, physical activity or body mass index (BMI) score [38].

6. Conclusions, Future Perspectives and Limitations

Here, in this review, we explored evidence of how exposure to high-sugar diets can contribute to the obese phenotype and lead to the development of NCDs later in life. In fact, it could be observed that an increased intake of dietary sugars during pregnancy, lactation, childhood and puberty are all risk factors for the development of cardiometabolic dysfunctions, with serious implications for aging, as shown in Figure 1.

It is evident that the DOHaD concept is gaining great notoriety around the world. Scientific societies and events have been organized with the aim of bringing together researchers and knowledge about how the first 1000 days after birth can be decisive throughout life, especially during aging. It has also been well known that sexual dimorphism is a factor that differentiates phenotypic responses throughout the critical phases of development. However, many gaps still need to be filled in order to better understand how perinatal life and puberty can be decisive for programming a healthy phenotype throughout life. It remains unknown how increased sugar intake during critical phases of development affects: (1) release of GnRH, which is mainly stimulated by kisspeptin; (2) the release of FSH and LH and their trophic effects on the gonads, and whether this differential release interferes with puberty onset; and (3) the ghrelin release and its actions on the CNS, as well as the release of GH, since blood glucose or dietary sugars interfere with the release of these two hormones. Finally, we hope that more experimental and cohort studies under the DOHaD concept can contribute to improving public policies and updating guidelines to provide recommendations about the risks of the intake of sugars, and can also contribute to elaborating interventions for improving healthy development.

The main limitation of this study is that, compared to other risk factors such as high-fat diet, relatively few studies have been dedicated to investigating the effects of dietary sugars during critical phases of development. Studies using animal models have demonstrated interesting results; however, the direct applicability of these protocols to humans is almost impossible. In this sense, more experimental studies are necessary to unravel late clinical interventions for mitigating the effects of early-life high sugar consumption or high glucose environment exposure.

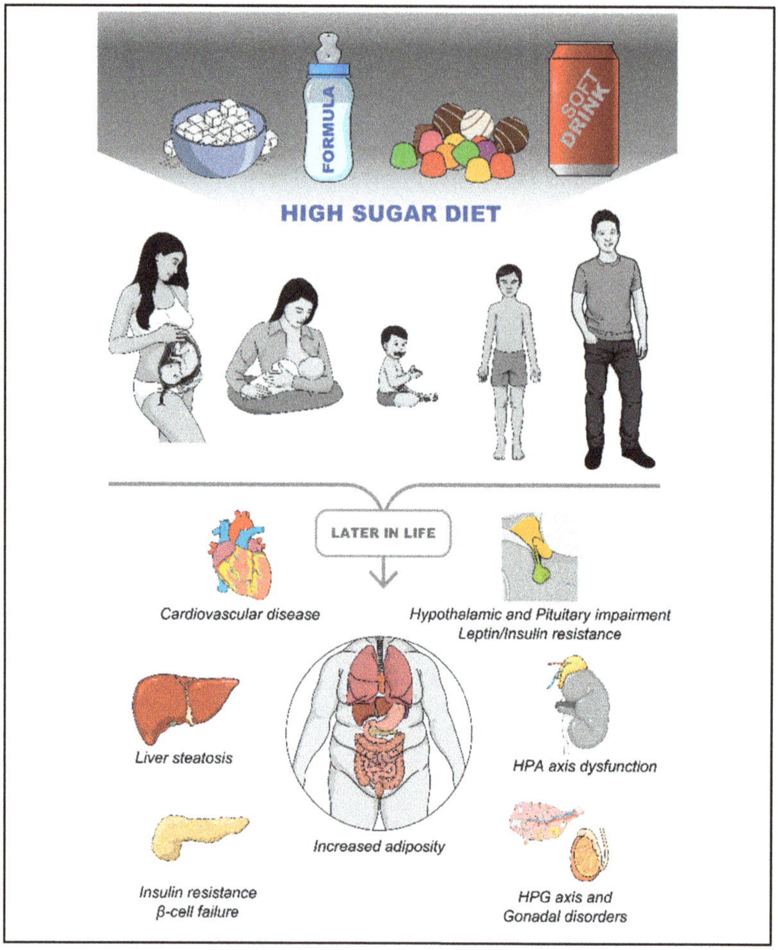

Figure 1. Schematic representation of how dietary sugars during critical phases of development affect healthy development, leading to an obese phenotype in adulthood, with many dysfunctions of homeostasis.

Author Contributions: Conceptualization, R.M.G.; methodology, R.M.G. and M.D.F.-J.; investigation, M.D.F.-J., K.V.N.C. and A.P.C.d.M.; writing—original draft preparation, M.D.F.-J., K.V.N.C., A.P.C.d.M. and R.M.G.; writing—review and editing, M.D.F.-J.; funding acquisition, R.M.G. All authors have read and agreed to the published version of the manuscript.

Funding: Funding was provided by the Conselho Nacional de Desenvolvimento Científico e Tecnológico (CNPq) (grant number 405712/2021-9), Coordenação de Aperfeiçoamento de Pessoal de Nível Superior (CAPES) (Finance code 001).

Institutional Review Board Statement: Not applicable.

Informed Consent Statement: Not applicable.

Data Availability Statement: Not applicable.

Conflicts of Interest: The authors declare no conflict of interest.

References

1. World Health Organization. *Taking Action on Childhood Obesity*; World Health Organization: Geneva, Switzerland, 2018; pp. 1–8.
2. Ferreira, L.; Ferreira-Junior, M.; Amaral, K.; Cavalcante, K.; Pontes, C.; Ribeiro, L.; Santos, B.G.D.; Xavier, C.H.; de Freitas Mathias, P.C.; Andersen, M.L.; et al. Maternal postnatal early overfeeding induces sex-related cardiac dysfunction and alters sexually hormones levels in young offspring. *J. Nutr. Biochem.* **2022**, *103*, 108969. [CrossRef]
3. Grilo, L.F.; Tocantins, C.; Diniz, M.S.; Gomes, R.M.; Oliveira, P.J.; Matafome, P.; Pereira, S.P. Metabolic Disease Programming: From Mitochondria to Epigenetics, Glucocorticoid Signalling and Beyond. *Eur. J. Clin. Investig.* **2021**, *51*, e13625. [CrossRef]
4. Langley-Evans, S.C.; McMullen, S. Developmental Origins of Adult Disease. *Med. Princ. Prac.* **2010**, *19*, 87–98. [CrossRef]
5. Lacagnina, S. The Developmental Origins of Health and Disease (DOHaD). *Am. J. Lifestyle Med.* **2020**, *14*, 47–50. [CrossRef]
6. Menzo, E.L.; Cappellani, A.; Zanghì, A.; Di Vita, M.; Berretta, M.; Szomstein, S. Nutritional Implications of Obesity: Before and After Bariatric Surgery. *Bariatr. Surg. Prac. Patient Care* **2014**, *9*, 9–17. [CrossRef]
7. World Health Organization. *Guideline: Sugars Intake for Adults and Children*; World Health Organization: Geneva, Switzerland, 2015.
8. Wu, X.; Cui, L.; Wang, H.; Xu, J.; Zhong, Z.; Jia, X.; Wang, J.; Zhang, H.; Shi, Y.; Tang, Y.; et al. Impact of dietary sucralose and sucrose-sweetened water intake on lipid and glucose metabolism in male mice. *Eur. J. Nutr.* **2022**, *62*, 199–211. [CrossRef]
9. Veit, M.; van Asten, R.; Olie, A.; Prinz, P. The role of dietary sugars, overweight, and obesity in type 2 diabetes mellitus: A narrative review. *Eur. J. Clin. Nutr.* **2022**, *76*, 1497–1501. [CrossRef]
10. Aragno, M.; Mastrocola, R. Dietary Sugars and Endogenous Formation of Advanced Glycation Endproducts: Emerging Mechanisms of Disease. *Nutrients* **2017**, *9*, 385. [CrossRef]
11. Francisco, F.A.; Saavedra, L.P.J.; Junior, M.D.F.; Barra, C.; Matafome, P.; Mathias, P.C.F.; Gomes, R.M. Early AGEing and metabolic diseases: Is perinatal exposure to glycotoxins programming for adult-life metabolic syndrome? *Nutr. Rev.* **2021**, *79*, 13–24. [CrossRef]
12. Begdache, L.; Sadeghzadeh, S.; Pearlmutter, P.; Derose, G.; Krishnamurthy, P.; Koh, A. Dietary Factors, Time of the Week, Physical Fitness and Saliva Cortisol: Their Modulatory Effect on Mental Distress and Mood. *Int. J. Environ. Res. Public Health* **2022**, *19*, 7001. [CrossRef]
13. Maslova, E.; Halldorsson, T.I.; Astrup, A.; Olsen, S.F. Dietary protein-to-carbohydrate ratio and added sugar as determinants of excessive gestational weight gain: A prospective cohort study. *BMJ Open* **2015**, *5*, e005839. [CrossRef]
14. Renault, K.M.; Carlsen, E.M.; Nørgaard, K.; Nilas, L.; Pryds, O.; Secher, N.J.; Olsen, S.F.; Halldórsson, T.I. Intake of Sweets, Snacks and Soft Drinks Predicts Weight Gain in Obese Pregnant Women: Detailed Analysis of the Results of a Randomised Controlled Trial. *PLoS ONE* **2015**, *10*, e0133041. [CrossRef]
15. Jen, K.-L.C.; Rochon, C.; Zhong, S.; Whitcomb, L. Fructose and Sucrose Feeding during Pregnancy and Lactation in Rats Changes Maternal and Pup Fuel Metabolism. *J. Nutr.* **1991**, *121*, 1999–2005. [CrossRef]
16. Arima, Y.; Fukuoka, H. Developmental origins of health and disease theory in cardiology. *J. Cardiol.* **2020**, *76*, 14–17. [CrossRef]
17. Munetsuna, E.; Yamada, H.; Yamazaki, M.; Ando, Y.; Mizuno, G.; Hattori, Y.; Sadamoto, N.; Ishikawa, H.; Ohta, Y.; Fujii, R.; et al. Maternal high-fructose intake increases circulating corticosterone levels via decreased adrenal corticosterone clearance in adult offspring. *J. Nutr. Biochem.* **2019**, *67*, 44–50. [CrossRef]
18. Rodrigo, S.; Fauste, E.; de la Cuesta, M.; Rodríguez, L.; Álvarez-Millán, J.J.; Panadero, M.I.; Otero, P.; Bocos, C. Maternal fructose induces gender-dependent changes in both LXRα promoter methylation and cholesterol metabolism in progeny. *J. Nutr. Biochem.* **2018**, *61*, 163–172. [CrossRef]
19. Rodríguez, L.; Panadero, M.I.; Roglans, N.; Otero, P.; Álvarez-Millán, J.J.; Laguna, J.C.; Bocos, C. Fructose during pregnancy affects maternal and fetal leptin signaling. *J. Nutr. Biochem.* **2013**, *24*, 1709–1716. [CrossRef]
20. Vickers, M.H.; Clayton, Z.E.; Yap, C.; Sloboda, D.M. Maternal Fructose Intake during Pregnancy and Lactation Alters Placental Growth and Leads to Sex-Specific Changes in Fetal and Neonatal Endocrine Function. *Endocrinology* **2011**, *152*, 1378–1387. [CrossRef]
21. Grove, K.L.; Grayson, B.E.; Glavas, M.M.; Xiao, X.Q.; Smith, M.S. Development of metabolic systems. *Physiol. Behav.* **2005**, *86*, 646–660. [CrossRef]
22. Ahima, R.S.; Prabakaran, D.; Flier, J.S. Postnatal leptin surge and regulation of circadian rhythm of leptin by feeding. Implications for energy homeostasis and neuroendocrine function. *J. Clin. Investig.* **1998**, *101*, 1020–1027. [CrossRef]
23. World Health Organization; UNICEF. *WHO | Global Strategy for Infant and Young Child Feeding*; WHO: Geneva, Switzerland, 2017; Volume 53, pp. 1–5. Available online: http://apps.who.int/gb/archive/pdf_files/WHA54/ea54id4.pdf?ua=1&ua=1 (accessed on 1 May 2023).
24. Borba, V.V.; McGonagle, D.; Shoenfeld, Y. Breastfeeding and autoimmunity: Programing health from the beginning. *Am. J. Reprod. Immunol.* **2018**, *79*, e12778. [CrossRef]
25. Plagemann, A.; Harder, T.; Schellong, K.; Schulz, S.; Stupin, J.H. Early postnatal life as a critical time window for determination of long-term metabolic health. *Best Prac. Res. Clin. Endocrinol. Metab.* **2012**, *26*, 641–653. [CrossRef]
26. Gomes, R.M.; Bueno, F.G.; Schamber, C.R.; de Mello, J.C.P.; de Oliveira, J.C.; Francisco, F.A.; Moreira, V.M.; Junior, M.D.F.; Pedrino, G.R.; Mathias, P.C.D.F.; et al. Maternal diet-induced obesity during suckling period programs offspring obese phenotype and hypothalamic leptin/insulin resistance. *J. Nutr. Biochem.* **2018**, *61*, 24–32. [CrossRef]

27. Berger, P.K.; Plows, J.F.; Jones, R.B.; Alderete, T.L.; Rios, C.; Pickering, T.A.; Fields, D.A.; Bode, L.; Peterson, B.S.; Goran, M.I. Associations of maternal fructose and sugar-sweetened beverage and juice intake during lactation with infant neurodevelopmental outcomes at 24 months. *Am. J. Clin. Nutr.* **2020**, *112*, 1516–1522. [CrossRef]
28. Francisco, F.A.; Barella, L.F.; Silveira, S.D.S.; Saavedra, L.P.J.; Prates, K.V.; Alves, V.S.; Franco, C.C.D.S.; Miranda, R.A.; Ribeiro, T.A.; Tófolo, L.P.; et al. Methylglyoxal treatment in lactating mothers leads to type 2 diabetes phenotype in male rat offspring at adulthood. *Eur. J. Nutr.* **2018**, *57*, 477–486. [CrossRef]
29. Peppa, M.; He, C.; Hattori, M.; McEvoy, R.; Zheng, F.; Vlassara, H. Fetal or Neonatal Low-Glycotoxin Environment Prevents Autoimmune Diabetes in NOD Mice. *Diabetes* **2003**, *52*, 1441–1448. [CrossRef]
30. Rose, C.; Birch, L.L.; Savage, J.S. Dietary patterns in infancy are associated with child diet and weight outcomes at 6 years. *Int. J Obes.* **2017**, *41*, 783–788. [CrossRef]
31. Weijs, P.J.; Kool, L.M.; van Baar, N.M.; van der Zee, S.C. High beverage sugar as well as high animal protein intake at infancy may increase overweight risk at 8 years: A prospective longitudinal pilot study. *Nutr. J.* **2011**, *10*, 95. [CrossRef]
32. Tohi, M.; Bay, J.L.; Tu'akoi, S.; Vickers, M.H. The Developmental Origins of Health and Disease: Adolescence as a Critical Lifecourse Period to Break the Transgenerational Cycle of NCDs—A Narrative Review. *Int. J. Environ. Res. Public Health* **2022**, *19*, 6024. [CrossRef]
33. U.S. Department of Agriculture; U.S. Department of Health and Human Services. *Dietary Guidelines for Americans, 2020–2025*, 9th ed.; U.S. Department of Health and Human Services: Washington, DC, USA, 2020.
34. Harrell, C.; Zainaldin, C.; McFarlane, D.; Hyer, M.; Stein, D.; Sayeed, I.; Neigh, G. High-fructose diet during adolescent development increases neuroinflammation and depressive-like behavior without exacerbating outcomes after stroke. *Brain Behav. Immun.* **2018**, *73*, 340–351. [CrossRef]
35. Béghin, L.; Huybrechts, I.; Drumez, E.; Kersting, M.; Walker, R.W.; Kafatos, A.; Molnar, D.; Manios, Y.; Moreno, L.A.; De Henauw, S.; et al. High Fructose Intake Contributes to Elevated Diastolic Blood Pressure in Adolescent Girls: Results from The HELENA Study. *Nutrients* **2021**, *13*, 3608. [CrossRef]
36. Schwimmer, J.B.; Ugalde-Nicalo, P.; Welsh, J.A.; Angeles, J.E.; Cordero, M.; Harlow, K.E.; Alazraki, A.; Durelle, J.; Knight-Scott, J.; Newton, K.P.; et al. Effect of a Low Free Sugar Diet vs Usual Diet on Nonalcoholic Fatty Liver Disease in Adolescent Boys. *JAMA* **2019**, *321*, 256–265. [CrossRef]
37. Welsh, J.A.; Sharma, A.; Cunningham, S.; Vos, M.B. Consumption of Added Sugars and Indicators of Cardiovascular Disease Risk Among US Adolescents. *Circulation* **2011**, *123*, 249–257. [CrossRef]
38. Rodríguez, L.A.; Madsen, K.A.; Cotterman, C.; Lustig, R.H. Added sugar intake and metabolic syndrome in US adolescents: Cross-sectional analysis of the National Health and Nutrition Examination Survey 2005–2012. *Public Health Nutr.* **2016**, *19*, 2424–2434. [CrossRef]

diabetology

Systematic Review

The Impact of Moderate-to-High-Intensity Exercise Protocols on Glycated Hemoglobin Levels in Type 2 Diabetes Patients

Ana Pedrosa [1,2,*], Guilherme Furtado [1,3,*], Marcelo Paes de Barros [4], André Luís Lacerda Bachi [5], José Pedro Ferreira [1], Vilma A. Sardão [2,6], Luís Rama [1] and Ana Teixeira [1]

1 Faculty of Sport Sciences and Physical Education (FCDEF-UC), University of Coimbra-Research Unit for Sport and Physical Activity (CIDAF, UID/PTD/04213/2020), 3040-256 Coimbra, Portugal
2 CNC-Center for Neuroscience and Cell Biology, CIBB-Centre for Innovative Biomedicine and Biotechnology, University of Coimbra, 3004-504 Coimbra, Portugal
3 Polytechnic Institute of Coimbra, Applied Research Institute, Rua da Misericórdia, Lagar dos Corticos–S. Martinho do Bispo, 3045-093 Coimbra, Portugal
4 Institute of Physical Activity Sciences and Sports (ICAFE), MSc/PhD Interdisciplinary Program in Health Sciences, Cruzeiro do Sul University, São Paulo 01506-000, Brazil
5 Post-Graduation Program in Health Sciences, Santo Amaro University (UNISA), São Paulo 04829-300, Brazil
6 Multidisciplinary Institute of Aging (MIA Portugal), University of Coimbra, 3004-504 Coimbra, Portugal
* Correspondence: anapedrosa90@gmail.com (A.P.); guilhermefurtado@ipc.pt (G.F.)

Abstract: Type 2 diabetes mellitus (T2DM) is a growing global health issue that is closely linked to the epidemic of obesity. In addition to genetic factors, environmental and health-risk behaviours (i.e., high-carbohydrate diet and physical inactivity) contribute to a variety of pathophysiological disorders. Advanced exercise protocols, such as Moderate-to-intensity (MIT) and High Intensity Interval Training (HIIT), revealed a strategy for mitigating and/or attenuating the DTMII's harmful effects by controlling glycated haemoglobin (HbA1c) levels. The goals of this review were to summarize the most recent evidence on the impact of HIIT on HbA1c levels. A mini-review protocol was performed through the PubMed/Medline database. The search comprised experimental and randomized controlled trial studies published in English between 2016 and 2021. The terms HbA1c, T2DM, MIT and HIIT, and their analogues were used. A total of seven studies were finally included. Our findings showed that the HIIT protocol is an effective strategy to induce HbA1c balance and improve glycaemic control than moderate training. The HIIT conducted in the laboratory and involving aerobic exercise on a cycle ergometer appears to be more efficient that MIT. Additional findings include improved beta-cell function, decreased low-grade inflammation, and the induction of cardiovascular benefits. More research is required to investigate the feasibility and safety of HIIT protocols in T2DM patients.

Keywords: type 2 diabetes; exercise; glycated haemoglobin; blood glucose; nutrition

Citation: Pedrosa, A.; Furtado, G.; de Barros, M.P.; Bachi, A.L.L.; Ferreira, J.P.; Sardão, V.A.; Rama, L.; Teixeira, A. The Impact of Moderate-to-High-Intensity Exercise Protocols on Glycated Hemoglobin Levels in Type 2 Diabetes Patients. *Diabetology* **2023**, *4*, 11–18. https://doi.org/10.3390/diabetology4010002

Academic Editor: Paulo Matafome

Received: 12 November 2022
Revised: 17 December 2022
Accepted: 21 December 2022
Published: 28 December 2022

1. Introduction

The increase in type 2 diabetes mellitus (T2DM is an expanding global health problem closely linked to the epidemic of obesity [1]. This problem is considered a severe public health problem in terms of human life and average life expectancy [2]. In recent years, there has been an incidence increase, affecting individuals of all ages. The global burden of T2DM on people 20–79 years old is projected to increase to 629 million in 2045 compared to 425 million in 2017 [3]. T2DM is a metabolic disturbance characterized by a high level of sugar (glucose) in the blood, and it can cause symptoms such as excessive thirst, increase urination, and tiredness [4]. The body cannot use energy intake from food properly. The pancreas produces insulin, but it produces less over time, and cells resist insulin, resulting in insulin resistance metabolic syndrome [5]. Furthermore, individuals with this illness are at high risk for both micro- and macrovascular complications, such as retinopathy, nephropathy, and neuropathy [1]. Insulin deficiency also invariably leads to chronic hyperglycaemia, causing disturbances in carbohydrate, fat, and protein metabolism [6].

Insulin is a hormone produced by the pancreas, responsible for transporting the glucose in the bloodstream into the cells to be converted into energy [7]. A lack of insulin or the inability of cells to respond to its transport leads to hyperglycemia and the absence of glucose within the cell to perform its functions in the body [6,8]. The pancreatic β-cells are responsible for insulin production, synthesized as pre-proinsulin [9]. β-cell dysfunction is initially characterized by an impairment of insulin secretion during glucose stimulation and may occur before the inception of glucose intolerance in T2DM [10]. This dysfunction is characterized by a complex network of interactions between environmental factors such as obesity, an unhealthy diet, physical inactivity, and genetic factors that lead to multiple pathophysiological disturbances responsible for impaired glucose homeostasis in T2DM [2].

Both genetic and environmental factors significantly contribute to the multiple pathophysiological disturbances that cause impaired glucose homeostasis in type 2 diabetes. A high carbohydrate diet and sedentary lifestyle are the major factors for the rapidly increasing incidence of DM in developing countries [11]. Excessive fast sugar consumption and sedentary habits frequently result in hyperglycemia and hyperlipidemia, which can promote insulin resistance and chronic inflammation [12]. T2DM elevated glycated hemoglobin (HbA1c) level has recently been considered one the major risk factors for developing microvascular and macrovascular complications [1]. HbA1c is widely regarded as the gold standard for monitoring glycemic control and as a predictor of diabetes-related illnesses [13]. A decreased HbA1c level can be achieved through diet management [11], with recent research demonstrating the health benefits of regular exercise combined (or not) with a healthy diet in the balance of HbA1c [14]. A recent study observed that people who were inactive for more than 5–8 h a day had an average of 28% increased risk of T2DM [15].

Several studies indicated that regular exercise training has a positive impact on glucose homeostasis [16]. This impact is associated with a release of counter-regulatory hormones, training condition, and whether exercise was performed in the postabsorptive or the postprandial state. Nonetheless, the energy equivalent on exercise seems to represent the major determinant on changes in glucose homeostasis [17]. So, a single exercise training can increase the insulin sensibility by more than 48 h until recuperation, but this impact is relative to the intensity, duration, and type of exercise [18]. Traditional exercise guidelines have emphasized increasing moderate-to-intensity exercise training (MIT), with a minimum of 150 min week or 5 days/week of 30 min (i.e., with walking, jogging, cycling, muscle strength) in sedentary people [19], including the subgroups of T2DM patients [18]. Unlike LMPA, which requires staying in intervals of 40–60% of maximal aerobic capacity [19]. HIIT involves alternating between periods of vigorous exercise (defined as 70% maximum aerobic capacity) and periods of rest or recovery [18]. HIIT protocol positively impacts insulin resistance markers. This effect occurs from a metabolic adaptation resulting in a reduction of body fat and perhaps higher membrane-bound Glut-4 translocation [16].

In general, both MIT and HIIT protocols were linked to an increase in the insulin receptor phosphorylation at threonine G12, AKT phosphorylation at serin 473, and oxidative capacity in skeletal muscle increase [20]. Additionally, the increase in protein activities associated with glucose uptake, AMPK, CaMKII, and PGC1-α, improving insulin sensitivity, and glycemic marker of HbA1c were observed [20]. In fact, exercise has been shown to have clinical benefits such as improved insulin sensitivity, reduced HbA1c, and increased peak oxygen consumption, which are preventative of diabetes [21]. Furthermore, a growing body of literature has examined HIIT protocols but has not specifically focused on this marker. The present study aimed to review the impact of different types of exercise on HbA1c in patients with T2DM.

2. Materials and Methods

This mini systematic review (MSR) was guided by using the adapted version of Preferred Reporting Items for Systematic Review guidelines [22], and the previous published

MSR statement [23]. The search strategies were developed by three authors (A.P., G.E.F., and J.P.F.). For the final study selection, the following criteria were used: (i) randomized control trials carried out on T2DM patients of both sexes over 18 years old; (ii) studies with reported quantitative or calculable HbA1c before and after the exercise intervention. We excluded studies that did not report pre-DM and type 1 DM conditions, did not present an exercise intervention, and did not measure HbA1c before and after the exercise protocol. The searches were conducted between December 2021 and February 2022. Only papers in the English language were included. The study search strategies were centered on three indexed Medical Subject Heading (MeSH) concepts and their similarities. These concepts were used to restrict the obtained results to those related to humans due to our group desire to conduct future research on this population Table 1. The PICO (participants, intervention, comparison, and outcomes) framework was used to characterize each study of this MSR [24].

Table 1. Strategy of meta-search using MeSH terms and PICO guidelines.

Acronym	Information	Concepts	MeSH Terms
P	T2DM patients	People diagnosed with type II diabetes, which causes insulin resistance, among other symptoms	"Diabetes Mellitus, Type 2" OR/AND "Type 2 Diabetes"
I	HIIT	A type of exercise proocol that involves moderate continuos and/or alternating between periods of vigorous exercise and rest or recovery	"exercise" OR/AND "exercise therapy" OR/AND "moderate exercise" OR/AND "High Intensity Interval training"
C	T2DM patients	Without a specific treatment and/or involving isolated or combined physical exercise.	-
O	Hb1C	Reflects erythrocytes' cumulative glucose exposure over a time period proportional to erythrocyte survival.	"Glycated hemoglobin" AND Glycated human hemoglobin"

Notes: MIT = Moderate-to-intensity training; HIIT = High intensity interval training; T2DM = type 2 diabetes mellitus; Hb1C = glycated hemoglobin; PICO = participants, intervention, comparison, and outcomes.

3. Results

3.1. Identifying Eligible Studies

During the article search, 73 articles were found in the PubMed database and imported into the Endnote reference manager, which found no duplication. Following the title selection, 41 articles were eliminated for the following reasons: (i) other diseases than diabetes type 2, (ii) supplementation; (iii) under 18 years of age. Following a review of the abstracts, 14 articles were eliminated for the following reasons: (i) there was no control group; (ii) there was no exercise program; (iii) reviews; and (iv) an animal model was used. Finally, seven articles were chosen for this MSR.

3.2. General Characteristics of Studies

The studies chosen included interventions in women and men over 50 years old with T2DM, with a sample size ranging from 11 to 265 participants [25–31]. The body mass index of participants ranged from 23 to 40 kg/m^2, and they were diagnosed with T2DM within 4 years. All included articles measured HbA1c, before and after the exercise intervention. High-intensity interval training (HIIT, 3 studies) [25,29,31], high-intensity progressive resistance training (PRT, 1 study) [26], endurance training (END, 2 studies) [30,31], high-intensity interval training combined with resistance training (HIIT+RT, 1 study) [28], moderate-intensity training combined with resistance training (MCT+RT, 1 study) [28], and endurance training combined with resistance training (END+RT, 1 study) [27] were the different types of training protocols found, as shown in Table 2. The intervention time varies between two weeks and twelve months. Of all the selected studies, three studies include a control group without exercise [25–27], two studies compare two different protocols of exercise [28,31], and two studies compare the impact of exercise pre- and post-meals [29,30]. The study participants' ages are quite similar, indicating that the studies focus was on middle-to-older-aged adults. In general, all types of exercise positively impact HbA1c, but the studies involving a HIIT protocol presented more promising results [25,26,28,29,31].

Table 2. Summary of included studies according PICO guidelines.

Author	Participants (Mean Age)	Description of Interventions	Comparison (Controls)	Outcome (HbA1c/mmol/mol)
Cassidy, S. et al. 2019 [25]	n = 22 60 years old	12 weeks, HIIT group: 36 cycle sessions (3 sessions/week). 1 week was 2 min, increasing 10 s each week.	No Exercise	Decreased on HIIT Group on HbA1c 54.4 ± 3.3 vs. 51.6 ± 3.2 compared no exercise group 55.0 ± 1.8 57.0 ± 2.3.
Hangping, Z. et al. 2019 [26]	n = 265 66 years old	1 training session/week, 5–10 min weekly, 4 exercises.	No Exercise	PRT protocol was more efficient 6.83 ± 1.31vs 6.75 ± 0.93, than no exercise group 6.92 ± 1. Vs. 6.85 ± 1.17.
Johansen, M. et al. 2020 [27]	n = 95 56 years old	12 months 5 or 6 aerobic exercise sessions/week, 2 or 3 sessions/week, combined with resistance exercise.	No Exercise	BG reduced in the END + RT, 48.7 (9.0) vs −3.3 (−5.0, −1.7) compared with the standard care group, 50.2 (9.6). vs. −0.5 (−2.7, 1.8).
Magalhães, J. et al. 2018 [28]	n = 80 59 years old	12 months, MCT–continuous cycling at 40 to 60% HRR, HIIT group, both groups complete RT 10–12 repetitions.	HIIT RT MCT RT	No interaction between the intervention groups, HIIT + RT Group 52.1 ± 9.6 vs. 52.8 ± 7.1, MCT + RCT Group 53.0 ± 17.4. vs. 54.0 ± 14.8, and control group 51.7 ± 11.7 vs. 54.8 ± 11.1, in glycemic variables.
Savikj, M. et al. 2019 [29]	n = 11 60 years old	Cycle ergometer: 7 min warm-up, 6 pulses of 1 min (220 W, range 180–350 W) 75 rpm. 2 weeks, 3 sessions/week.	Post-morning Post-afternoon	Afternoon HIIT 48.3 ± 3.9 vs. 46.1 ± 2.7, was better at improving BG, but post-Morning 48.3 ± 3.9 vs. 45.1 ± 2.1, was better on HbA1c reduction in post-morning intervention.
Verboven, K. et al. 2020 [30]	n = 25 61 years old	12-week endurance training (3 exercise sessions/week), 25 min—walking, 20 min cycling, 65% of baseline VO2peak.	Fasted state Fed state	HbA1c better improved with exercise performed in the postprandial period 6.6 [6.3–7.5] vs. 6.3 [6.0–6.9], than 7.4 [6.8–8.2] vs. 7.7 [6.7–8.3].
Winding, K. et al. 2018 [31]	n = 29 56 years old	11-week, on bicycle, 3 days/week. END—40 min/session at 50% of Wpeak, group. HIIT—20 min/session of 95% Wpeak.	END HIIT	HIIT Intervention 7.4 [6.8–8.2] vs 7.7 [6.7–8.3] a statistically significant difference was observed in the reduction of HbA1c, when compare bout group, END group 52.2 ± 10.1. vs 51.4 ± 8.8 and, no exercise group 53.2 ± 12.6 vs 51.8 ± 11.3

Notes: HIIT = high-intensity interval training; MCT = moderate-intensity training; HRR= heart rate reserve; RT = resistance training; END = endurance training; Con = control; MICT = moderate-intensity continuous training; eWLmax= estimated maximum workload; PRT = high-intensity progressive resistance training; ILG = intensive lifestyle group; BG = blood glucose.

3.3. Main Findings of the Studies

Comparing the different protocols applied, HIIT protocol showed a reduction in HbA1c. Low-volume HIIT exercise, typically involving less than 15 min of high-intensity exercise per session, can be safely implemented as a time-efficient exercise option for reducing blood glucose levels in individuals with, or at risk for, T2DM [18]. In the HIIT group, when compared to the control group (no exercise), the glycaemic control was improved, with a reduction in HbA1c [25]. Two studies presented the role of nutritional status during exercise, when comparing the moment of application of the HIIT protocol, in the afternoon (3 h later) or in the morning (1 h later). The HIIT exercise practice in the afternoon was more efficacious at improving blood glucose, but the HbA1c levels had increased reductions in the post-morning intervention [29]. These results indicated that the glucose intolerance, insulin sensitivity, and skeletal muscle oxidative capacity can fluctuate with circadian oscillations. The END exercise seemed to better improve HbA1c levels when performed in the postprandial period [30]. One study compared HIIT with MCT with RT with both groups presenting no differences in glycaemic control, but the MCT with RT improved the body composition and cardiorespiratory fitness [28]. Another study compared HIIT with END: the HIIT group reduced fasting glucose, HbA1c levels, and glycaemic variability, while the END group showed a reduction in gynoid fat mass and a tendency towards a reduction in whole body mass and visceral fat mass [31]. A PRT protocol showed a reduction in HbA1c at 6 months, improving glycaemic indices in elderly patients' adjunct to diet and medication [26]. Aerobic exercise combined with RT improved beta cell function, decreased low-grade inflammation and body weight, and reduced the HbA1c levels [27].

4. Discussion

Different exercise strategies demonstrate benefits for patients with T2DM, in terms of glycemic control, beta cell function, cardiovascular health and/or body weight. After our search through the recent literature, we observed that HIIT showed better results in reducing HbA1c than other (MCT, RT, END, MICT) exercise programs. In a study by Karstoft et al. [32], the impact of postprandial glycemic control and free-living glycemic control showed that HIIT had a greater impact in both variables than MICT. Our review confirms the results in the study of Savikj M. et al. 2019 [29], which showed that HIIT performed in the afternoon was better at improving blood glucose and HbA1c when compared to a post-morning intervention. Additionally, in the study by Verboven, K. et al. 2020 [30], HbA1c seems to be improved more with exercise performed in the postprandial period. In another study, Elsisi et al. 2015 [33] determined the impact of high-intensity interval training (HIIT) on glycated hemoglobin (HbA1c) in T2DM on a short-term basis (after 12 weeks of training), the results showing that HIIT was more effective and an alternative to aerobic training in improving HbA1c in T2DM. This confirms the results presented by Winding, K. et al. 2018 [31] in which, with the HIIT intervention, a statistically significant difference was observed in the reduction in HbA1c.

The main finding of this MSR was that HIIT improves glucose control centers' ability to recruit more muscle fibers and rapidly deplete muscle glycogen levels, thereby promoting a greater increase in post-exercise muscle insulin sensitivity [18]. With an increase in post-exercise muscle insulin sensitivity between 24 and 48 h after a single exercise, HIIT may be an effective strategy to improve glucose control acutely and in the long term. A HIIT protocol for 12–16 weeks may show a positive impact on reducing abdominal fat and increasing lean muscle mass. This type of exercise recently assumed a prominent role in physical activity and health, showing cardiovascular and metabolic benefits in patients with chronic diseases, including T2DM [34–36]. However, the HIIT protocol may induce increases in VO_{2max} in patients with metabolic disorders and healthy individuals. This protocol also improves the change in the systolic volume of the heart, induced by increased cardiac contractility and the oxidative capacity of skeletal muscle, in addition to changes in glucose transport, which improve the mitochondrial function to generate more adenosine triphosphate, as well as increasing the aerobic capacity [37].

This MSR presented some limitations as the search was performed in one database and only included articles published within the last 5 years. This review focused on HbA1c as the ultimate measure of glycemic control due to the lack of studies regarding the impact of exercise on dietary sugars. Considering that physical exercise has a positive impact on T2DM patients, it would be interesting in the future to analyze the independent and combined effect of exercise on these variables in T2DM patients. A systematic review with meta-analysis can be future performed, controlling for the type of exercise, which represents the main publication bias in this type of work.

5. Conclusions

The exercise protocol of HIIT seems to be a more effective exercise strategy to improve HbA1c compared to other training protocols in middle-aged patients with T2DM. This type of exercise seems to be safe in these patients, but a pre-exercise clinical evaluation is necessary for its safe performance.

Author Contributions: A.P. and G.F. designed the study; A.P. collected the data, performed data analysis, and wrote the manuscript, G.F. provided guidance; G.F., J.P.F., M.P.d.B., A.L.L.B., A.T., V.A.S. and L.R. read and provided feedback on the manuscript. All authors read and approved the final version. All authors have read and agreed to the published version of the manuscript.

Funding: This research was funded by FCT—Fundação para a Ciência e a Tecnologia, grant number 2021. 07220.BD.

Institutional Review Board Statement: Not applicable.

Informed Consent Statement: Not applicable.

Data Availability Statement: Data is contained within the article.

Conflicts of Interest: The authors declare no conflict of interest.

References

1. De Fronzo, R.A.; Ferrannini, E.; Groop, L.; Henry, R.R.; Herman, W.H.; Holst, J.J.; Hu, F.B.; Kahn, C.R.; Raz, I.; Shulman, G.I.; et al. Type 2 diabetes mellitus. *Nat. Rev. Dis. Prim.* **2015**, *1*, 15019. [CrossRef] [PubMed]
2. Khan, M.A.B.; Hashim, M.J.; King, J.K.; Govender, R.D.; Mustafa, H.; Al Kaabi, J. Epidemiology of Type 2 Diabetes—Global Burden of Disease and Forecasted Trends. *J. Epidemiol. Glob. Health* **2020**, *10*, 107–111. [CrossRef] [PubMed]
3. Al-Rifai, R.H.; Majeed, M.; Qambar, M.A.; Ibrahim, A.; AlYammahi, K.M.; Aziz, F. Type 2 diabetes and pre-diabetes mellitus: A systematic review and meta-analysis of prevalence studies in women of childbearing age in the Middle East and North Africa, 2000–2018. *Syst. Rev.* **2019**, *8*, 268. [CrossRef]
4. Clinic, C. Type 2 Diabetes. 2021. Available online: https://my.clevelandclinic.org/health/diseases/21501-type-2-diabetes (accessed on 12 December 2022).
5. Wilcox, G. Insulin and insulin resistance. *Clin. Biochem. Rev.* **2005**, *26*, 19–39.
6. Chew, B.H.; Vos, R.C.; Metzendorf, M.I.; Scholten, R.J.; Rutten, G.E. Psychological interventions for diabetes-related distress in adults with type 2 diabetes mellitus. *Cochrane Database Syst. Rev.* **2017**, *9*. [CrossRef]
7. Rahman, M.S.; Hossain, K.S.; Das, S.; Kundu, S.; Adegoke, E.O.; Rahman, M.A.; Hannan, M.A.; Uddin, M.J.; Pang, M.G. Role of Insulin in Health and Disease: An Update. *Int. J. Mol. Sci.* **2021**, *22*, 6403. [CrossRef]
8. Santos, M.; West, E.; Skali, H.; Forman, D.E.; Nadruz, W.J.; Shah, A.M. Resting Heart Rate and Chronotropic Response to Exercise: Prognostic Implications in Heart Failure Across the Left Ventricular Ejection Fraction Spectrum. *J. Card Fail.* **2018**, *24*, 753–762. [CrossRef]
9. Galicia-Garcia, U.; Benito-Vicente, A.; Jebari, S.; Larrea-Sebal, A.; Siddiqi, H.; Uribe, K.B.; Ostolaza, H.; Martín, C. Pathophysiology of Type 2 Diabetes Mellitus. *Int. J. Mol. Sci.* **2020**, *21*, 6275. [CrossRef]
10. Klonoff, D.C.; Buckingham, B.; Christiansen, J.S.; Montori, V.M.; Tamborlane, W.V.; Vigersky, R.A.; Wolpert, H. Withdrawn as duplicate: Corrigendum to: Continuous Glucose Monitoring: An Endocrine Society Clinical Practice Guideline. *J. Clin. Endocrinol. Metab.* **2022**, *107*, e2220.
11. Sami, W.; Ansari, T.; Butt, N.S.; Hamid, M.R.A. Effect of diet on type 2 diabetes mellitus: A review. *Int. J. Health Sci.* **2017**, *11*, 65–71.
12. Galaviz, K.I.; Narayan, K.M.V.; Lobelo, F.; Weber, M.B. Lifestyle and the Prevention of Type 2 Diabetes: A Status Report. *Am. J. Lifestyle Med.* **2018**, *12*, 4–20. [CrossRef] [PubMed]

13. Niwaha, A.J.; Rodgers, L.R.; Greiner, R.; Balungi, P.A.; Mwebaze, R.; McDonald, T.J.; Hattersley, A.T.; Shields, B.M.; Nyirenda, M.J.; Jones, A.G. HbA1c performs well in monitoring glucose control even in populations with high prevalence of medical conditions that may alter its reliability: The OPTIMAL observational multicenter study. *BMJ Open Diabetes Res. Care* **2021**, *9*, e002350. [CrossRef] [PubMed]
14. Stephenson, E.J.; Smiles, W.; Hawley, J.A. The relationship between exercise, nutrition and type 2 diabetes. *Med. Sport Sci.* **2014**, *60*, 1–10. [PubMed]
15. Li, D.-D.; Yang, Y.; Gao, Z.-Y.; Zhao, L.-H.; Yang, X.; Xu, F.; Yu, C.; Zhang, X.-L.; Wang, X.-Q.; Wang, L.-H.; et al. Sedentary lifestyle and body composition in type 2 diabetes. *Diabetol. Metab. Syndr.* **2022**, *14*, 8. [CrossRef] [PubMed]
16. Santos, I.K.D.; Nunes, F.; Queiros, V.S.; Cobucci, R.N.; Dantas, P.B.; Soares, G.M.; Cabral, B.; Maranhão, T.M.O.; Dantas, P.M.S. Effect of high-intensity interval training on metabolic parameters in women with polycystic ovary syndrome: A systematic review and meta-analysis of randomized controlled trials. *PLoS ONE* **2021**, *16*, e0245023. [CrossRef]
17. Younk, L.M.; Mikeladze, M.; Tate, D.; Davis, S.N. Exercise-related hypoglycemia in diabetes mellitus. *Expert. Rev. Endocrinol. Metab.* **2011**, *6*, 93–108. [CrossRef]
18. Francois, M.E.; Little, J.P. Effectiveness and safety of high-intensity interval training in patients with type 2 diabetes. *Diabetes Spectr.* **2015**, *28*, 39–44. [CrossRef]
19. Colberg, S.R.; Sigal, R.J.; Fernhall, B.; Regensteiner, J.G.; Blissmer, B.J.; Rubin, R.R.; Chasan-Taber, L.; Albright, A.L.; Braun, B. Exercise and type 2 diabetes: The American College of Sports Medicine and the American Diabetes Association: Joint position statement. *Diabetes Care* **2010**, 33, e147–e167. [CrossRef]
20. Jiménez-Maldonado, A.; García-Suárez, P.C.; Rentería, I.; Moncada-Jiménez, J.; Plaisance, E.P. Impact of high-intensity interval training and sprint interval training on peripheral markers of glycemic control in metabolic syndrome and type 2 diabetes. *Biochim. Biophys. Acta Mol. Basis Dis.* **2020**, *1866*, 165820. [CrossRef]
21. Amanat, S.; Ghahri, S.; Dianatinasab, A.; Fararouei, M.; Dianatinasab, M. Exercise and Type 2 Diabetes. *Adv. Exp. Med. Biol.* **2020**, *1228*, 91–105.
22. Page, M.J.; McKenzie, J.E.; Bossuyt, P.M.; Boutron, I.; Hoffmann, T.C.; Mulrow, C.D.; Shamseer, L.; Tetzlaff, J.M.; Akl, E.A.; Brennan, S.E.; et al. The PRISMA 2020 statement: An updated guideline for reporting systematic reviews. *Syst. Rev.* **2021**, *10*, 89. [CrossRef] [PubMed]
23. Griffiths, P. Evidence informing practice: Introducing the mini-review. *Br. J. Community Nurs.* **2002**, *7*, 38–39. [CrossRef] [PubMed]
24. Eriksen, M.B.; Frandsen, T.F. The impact of patient, intervention, comparison, outcome (PICO) as a search strategy tool on literature search quality: A systematic review. *J. Med. Libr. Assoc.* **2018**, *106*, 420–431. [CrossRef] [PubMed]
25. Cassidy, S.; Vaidya, V.; Houghton, D.; Zalewski, P.; Seferovic, J.P.; Hallsworth, K.; MacGowan, G.A.; Trenell, M.I.; Jakovljevic, D.G. Unsupervised high-intensity interval training improves glycaemic control but not cardiovascular autonomic function in type 2 diabetes patients: A randomised controlled trial. *Diab. Vasc. Dis. Res.* **2019**, *16*, 69–76. [CrossRef] [PubMed]
26. Hangping, Z.; Xiaona, Q.; Qi, Z.; Qingchun, L.; Na, Y.; Lijin, J.; Siying, L.; Shuo, Z.; Xiaoming, Z.; Xiaoxia, L.; et al. The impact on glycemic control through progressive resistance training with bioDensity(TM) in Chinese elderly patients with type 2 diabetes: The PReTTy2 (Progressive Resistance Training in Type 2 Diabetes) Trial. *Diabetes Res. Clin. Pract.* **2019**, *150*, 64–71. [CrossRef] [PubMed]
27. Johansen, M.Y.; Karstoft, K.; MacDonald, C.S.; Hansen, K.B.; Ellingsgaard, H.; Hartmann, B.; Wewer Albrechtsen, N.J.; Vaag, A.A.; Holst, J.J.; Pedersen, B.K.; et al. Effects of an intensive lifestyle intervention on the underlying mechanisms of improved glycaemic control in individuals with type 2 diabetes: A secondary analysis of a randomised clinical trial. *Diabetologia* **2020**, *63*, 2410–2422. [CrossRef] [PubMed]
28. Magalhães, J.P.; Júdice, P.B.; Ribeiro, R.; Andrade, R.; Raposo, J.; Dores, H.; Bicho, M.; Sardinha, L.B. Effectiveness of high-intensity interval training combined with resistance training versus continuous moderate-intensity training combined with resistance training in patients with type 2 diabetes: A one-year randomized controlled trial. *Diabetes Obes. Metab.* **2019**, *21*, 550–559. [CrossRef] [PubMed]
29. Savikj, M.; Gabriel, B.M.; Alm, P.S.; Smith, J.; Caidahl, K.; Björnholm, M.; Fritz, T.; Krook, A.; Zierath, J.R.; Wallberg-Henriksson, H. Afternoon exercise is more efficacious than morning exercise at improving blood glucose levels in individuals with type 2 diabetes: A randomised crossover trial. *Diabetologia* **2019**, *62*, 233–237. [CrossRef]
30. Verboven, K.; Wens, I.; Vandenabeele, F.; Stevens, A.N.; Celie, B.; Lapauw, B.; Dendale, P.; Van Loon, L.J.C.; Calders, P.; Hansen, D. Impact of Exercise-Nutritional State Interactions in Patients with Type 2 Diabetes. *Med. Sci. Sports Exerc.* **2020**, *52*, 720–728. [CrossRef]
31. Winding, K.M.; Munch, G.W.; Iepsen, U.W.; Van Hall, G.; Pedersen, B.K.; Mortensen, S.P. The effect on glycaemic control of low-volume high-intensity interval training versus endurance training in individuals with type 2 diabetes. *Diabetes Obes. Metab.* **2018**, *20*, 1131–1139. [CrossRef]
32. Karstoft, K.; Winding, K.; Knudsen, S.H.; Nielsen, J.S.; Thomsen, C.; Pedersen, B.K.; Solomon, T.P. The effects of free-living interval-walking training on glycemic control, body composition, and physical fitness in type 2 diabetic patients: A randomized, controlled trial. *Diabetes Care* **2013**, *36*, 228–236. [CrossRef] [PubMed]
33. Elsisia, H.F.; Aneisb, Y.M.; Mounirc, K.M. Impact of high-intensity interval training on HbA1c in patients with type 2 diabetes mellitus. *Bull. Fac. Phys. Ther.* **2015**, *20*, 168–175. [CrossRef]

34. Cassidy, S.; Thoma, C.; Houghton, D.; Trenell, M.I. High-intensity interval training: A review of its impact on glucose control and cardiometabolic health. *Diabetologia* **2017**, *60*, 7–23. [CrossRef] [PubMed]
35. Gibala, M.J.; Little, J.P.; Macdonald, M.J.; Hawley, J.A. Physiological adaptations to low-volume, high-intensity interval training in health and disease. *J. Physiol.* **2012**, *590*, 1077–1084. [CrossRef]
36. Mendes, R.; Sousa, N.; Themudo-Barata, J.L.; Reis, V.M. High-Intensity Interval Training Versus Moderate-Intensity Continuous Training in Middle-Aged and Older Patients with Type 2 Diabetes: A Randomized Controlled Crossover Trial of the Acute Effects of Treadmill Walking on Glycemic Control. *Int. J. Env. Res. Public. Health* **2019**, *16*, 4163. [CrossRef] [PubMed]
37. de Mello, M.B.; Righi, N.C.; Schuch, F.B.; Signori, L.U.; da Silva, A.M.V. Effect of high-intensity interval training protocols on VO2max and HbA1c level in people with type 2 diabetes: A systematic review and meta-analysis. *Ann. Phys. Rehabil. Med.* **2022**, *65*, 101586. [CrossRef] [PubMed]

MDPI
St. Alban-Anlage 66
4052 Basel
Switzerland
Tel. +41 61 683 77 34
Fax +41 61 302 89 18
www.mdpi.com

Diabetology Editorial Office
E-mail: diabetology@mdpi.com
www.mdpi.com/journal/diabetology